Competing Risks

STATISTICS IN PRACTICE

Advisory Editors

Stephen Senn
University of Glasgow, UK

Marian Scott
University of Glasgow, UK

Peter Bloomfield
North Carolina State University, USA

Founding Editor

Vic Barnett
Nottingham Trent University, UK

Statistics in Practice is an important international series of texts which provide detailed coverage of statistical concepts, methods and worked case studies in specific fields of investigation and study.

With sound motivation and many worked practical examples, the books show in down-to-earth terms how to select and use an appropriate range of statistical techniques in a particular practical field within each title's special topic area.

The books provide statistical support for professionals and research workers across a range of employment fields and research environments. Subject areas covered include medicine and pharmaceutics; industry, finance and commerce; public services; the earth and environmental sciences, and so on.

The books also provide support to students studying statistical courses applied to the above areas. The demand for graduates to be equipped for the work environment has led to such courses becoming increasingly prevalent at universities and colleges.

It is our aim to present judiciously chosen and well-written workbooks to meet everyday practical needs. Feedback of views from readers will be most valuable to monitor the success of this aim.

A complete list of titles in this series appears at the end of the volume.

Competing Risks

A Practical Perspective

Melania Pintilie
Ontario Cancer Institute, Canada

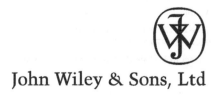

John Wiley & Sons, Ltd

Copyright © 2006   John Wiley & Sons Ltd, The Atrium, Southern Gate, Chichester,
West Sussex PO19 8SQ, England

Telephone   (+44) 1243 779777

Email (for orders and customer service enquiries): cs-books@wiley.co.uk
Visit our Home Page on www.wiley.com

Other Wiley Editorial Offices

John Wiley & Sons Inc., 111 River Street, Hoboken, NJ 07030, USA

Jossey-Bass, 989 Market Street, San Francisco, CA 94103-1741, USA

Wiley-VCH Verlag GmbH, Boschstr. 12, D-69469 Weinheim, Germany

John Wiley & Sons Australia Ltd, 42 McDougall Street, Milton, Queensland 4064, Australia

John Wiley & Sons (Asia) Pte Ltd, 2 Clementi Loop #02-01, Jin Xing Distripark, Singapore 129809

John Wiley & Sons Canada Ltd, 22 6045 Freemont Blvd, Mississauga, ONT, L5R 4J3

Wiley also publishes its books in a variety of electronic formats. Some content that appears in print may not be available in electronic books.

Library of Congress Cataloging in Publication Data

Pintilie, Melania.
    Competing risks : a practical perspective / Melania Pintilie.
        p.   cm.
    Includes bibliographical references and index.
    ISBN-13: 978-0-470-87068-6 (cloth : alk. paper)
    ISBN-10: 0-470-87068-0 (cloth : alk. paper)
    1. Competing risks.   I. Title.
    QA273.P485 2006
    519.2—dc22

                                    2006023988

British Library Cataloguing in Publication Data

A catalogue record for this book is available from the British Library

ISBN-13 978-0-470-87068-6 (HB)
ISBN-10 0-470-87068-0 (HB)

Typeset in 11/13pt Photina by Integra Software Services Pvt. Ltd, Pondicherry, India

What we have to learn to do, we learn by doing.

Aristotle

Contents

Preface

This book describes the methodology for the analysis of competing risks from the applied perspective. Although most of the examples are drawn from medical research, situations involving competing risks occur in many other areas, such as sociology, economics and engineering. Chapter 1 is a non-mathematical introduction to the topic of competing risks. The problems involved in the analysis of competing risks need to be understood by both the statistician and the scientist. Thus, this chapter gives enough detail to enable a meaningful discussion to take place between the scientist and the applied statistician. Some general techniques for survival analysis are included to facilitate the understanding of the theory of competing risks (Chapter 2). Chapters 3–6 cover the analysis of competing risks using nonparametric or semiparametric techniques. The sample size calculations under different scenarios are presented in Chapter 7. A brief overview of other aspects of the analysis of competing risks is included in Chapter 8, and examples are provided in Chapter 9 to complement the material in Chapter 1. Although Chapters 2–8 contain a certain amount of mathematical detail, an understanding of the concepts can be achieved through studying the examples given. For ease of exposition, subscripts are omitted whenever possible. Appendix A contains the mathematical proofs which were considered too elaborate to be included in the respective chapters. Details on how to perform the analyses are included in each chapter and are supplemented with R functions and SAS macros incorporated in Appendix B. For those readers who wish to extend their knowledge of the topic of competing risks, references to current theoretical developments are provided at the end of each chapter.

The datasets, the supplementary R functions and the SAS macros used in this book can be downloaded from

www.uhnresearch.ca/hypoxia/People_Pintilie.htm

I would be grateful to be informed of any errors, ambiguities or oversights found in this book.

Melania Pintilie
pintilie@uhnres.utoronto.ca

Acknowledgements

I would first like to express my warmest gratitude to Ellen Maki whose participation in shaping this book was crucial. Ellen contributed substantially to Chapters 2 and 4 and had many suggestions throughout. Richard Hill's help was invaluable. He thoroughly reviewed the material and generously shared his experience and expertise. I thank Janet Raboud for her careful reading and the highly competent advice she gave me. Richard and Janet's helpful comments contributed considerably to enhancing the clarity of the presentation of the material. I would also like to acknowledge the input given by Gina Lockwood and Ruth Croxford who kindly reviewed parts of this manuscript. Finally, I express my appreciation to the anonymous reviewers who read the manuscript and made many helpful comments and suggestions.

Special thanks go to Tony Panzarella who, as the manager of the Biostatistics Department of the Princess Margaret Hospital/Ontario Cancer Institute, reviewed the work and encouraged this endeavour from its earliest stages. The datasets used were from the Princess Margaret Hospital, a leading cancer centre in North America. I appreciate the generosity of the researchers, Mary Gospodarowicz, Anthony Fyles and Hans Messner, who graciously agreed to let me use their datasets as examples.

It was a pleasure to work with the team at Wiley, notably Rob Calver, who sowed the seeds for this book, and Kathryn Sharples, Simon Lightfoot and Wendy Hunter, who diligently helped me accomplish this project.

Last, but not least, I wish to thank my husband, Alex, whose help and support gave me the necessary confidence to continue.

1

Introduction

1.1 HISTORICAL NOTES

In the middle of the seventeenth century John Graunt, a haberdasher by trade, started to collect and tabulate the information included in the Bills of Mortality published weekly at that time in London. This work, probably done in collaboration with Sir William Petty, appeared in 1662 and contained a demographic summary of causes of death in England and Wales. As a result, John Graunt was elected a member of the Royal Society at the recommendation of King Charles II, not a small feat considering the hierarchical structure of the society existent at the time. In 1693, the famous astronomer, Edmund Halley, developed the concept of life tables in a format not unlike that used today in survival analysis. His data were based on the register of births and deaths for the city of Breslau (now Wrocław, in southwestern Poland). In 1760 Daniel Bernoulli applied Halley's method to demonstrate the advantages of smallpox inoculation. He calculated the increase in Halley's survivor function if smallpox were eliminated as a cause of death. In this way, Bernoulli founded the theory of competing risks. A summary of his work on competing risks can be found in David and Moeschberger (1978). From the eighteenth century, mathematics developed, notations changed and statistics branched out as a science in its own right. The great discoveries of the nineteenth century in physics and biology led to a deterministic

Competing Risks: A Practical Perspective   M. Pintilie
© 2006 John Wiley & Sons, Ltd

view of the universe. However, as the tools for measurement grew more and more precise it became apparent that some unexplained, random factors were at work. In the twentieth century, due in part to the need to explain the random variation and in part to the extraordinary development of computing capabilities, the theory of statistics saw significant progress. Based on Bernoulli's work, the theory of competing risks, referred to in actuarial sciences as *multiple decrements,* has also developed.

1.2   DEFINING COMPETING RISKS

This chapter presents an introduction to the topic of competing risks. It is intended for statisticians who have not had any exposure to competing risks and for non-statisticians whose research involves time-to-event data. The analysis of such data is usually referred to as *survival analysis,* because the theory was developed using death as the event. It is also called the *analysis of incomplete data.* The term *incomplete* refers to records where an event has not been observed, but is bound to take place if followed long enough. This type of observation is called *censored* and its definition can be found in Chapter 2. The event need not be death. It can be any event that occurs over time, such as relapse of disease, recidivism or discharge from hospital. Survival techniques are well developed and implemented in major statistical software. Yet, there are some situations where it may not be appropriate to apply the usual survival methods to the time-to-event analysis. One such situation is where competing risks are present. The competing risks situation can be defined in several different ways, as shown in Chapter 3. In general, a competing risks situation arises when an individual can experience more than one type of event and the occurrence of one type of event hinders the occurrence of other types of events. To illustrate this definition, suppose that a group of patients diagnosed with heart disease is followed in order to observe a myocardial infarction (MI). If by the end of the study each patient was either observed to have MI or was alive and well, then the usual survival techniques can be applied. In real life, however, some patients may die from other causes before experiencing an MI. This is a competing risks situation because death from other causes prohibits the occurrence of MI. MI is considered the event of interest, while death from other causes is considered a competing risk. The group of patients dead of other causes cannot be considered censored, since their observations are not incomplete.

1.3   USE OF THE KAPLAN–MEIER METHOD IN THE PRESENCE OF COMPETING RISKS

In the presence of competing risks, the usual survival methods should be applied with caution and one has to be aware of the consequences of their use. The Kaplan–Meier method is the most
  common as well as the most controversial technique in the competing risks framework. It is a method for estimating survival probabilities (Kaplan and Meier, 1958) at different time points. It is relatively easy to apply and interpret and can be depicted visually. Its wide availability in the statistical software makes its use appealing. When competing risks are present, Kaplan–Meier estimates (denoted by *KM*) cannot be interpreted as probabilities. Their complement $(1 - KM)$ can be interpreted as the probability of an event of interest in an ideal world where the other types of events do not exist. However, this concept is not useful in practice. Kalbfleisch and Prentice (1980) suggested an approach that accounted for the competing risks. This method is labelled the *cumulative incidence function* (CIF, introduced in Chapter 4). Using this technique, the probability of any event happening is partitioned into the probabilities for each type of event. For example, in the hypoxia trial described in Section 1.6.2, the possible events are local relapse (L), concomitant local and distant relapse (L&D) and distant relapse only (D). Usually death is a competing risk event. However, in this dataset, at the time of the analysis, there were no deaths without a local or distant relapse. The probability of *any* type of event occurring can be estimated using the Kaplan–Meier method $(1 - KM)$. The probability of *one* type of event is estimated using the CIF. At any point in time, $1 - KM$, calculated for all events, is equal to the sum of the cumulative incidence for each type of event. In Figure 1.1 the dashed line represents the cumulative incidence for events of type L only, and the thin solid line represents the CIF for L in addition to L&D. Therefore, the portion in between the first

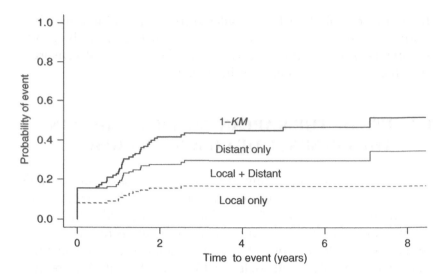

Figure 1.1 Partition of the complement of the Kaplan–Meier estimate $(1 - KM)$ into the three cumulative incidence functions – local, local and distant, and distant only – in the hypoxia trial.

and second lines is the probability of L&D. If the probability of D is added then the probability of any event is obtained, depicted as the solid thicker line.

In the presence of competing risks, $1 - KM$ does not estimate the probability of the occurrence of a type of event. To illustrate this idea, consider that the group of heart disease patients described earlier contains 20 individuals and they all either experienced an MI or died of other causes. The time and type of failure are given in Table 1.1. The time is given in months and the type of failure is coded as MI or D, the latter being used if the patient died of other causes. It is obvious that by 16 months 50% of the patients experienced MI. The cumulative incidence for MI at 16 months (calculated as shown in Chapter 4) is also 50%. However, the $1 - KM$ estimate at 16 months is 84%. Furthermore, $1 - KM$ for the competing risks (for D) at 16 months is 100%. If we interpret $1 - KM$ as the probability of the event occurring by a certain time t, then the sum of the value of $1 - KM$ for MI and the value for $1 - KM$ for D gives the probability that any of these events happened by time t. In this case, the $1 - KM$ estimates at 16 months are 0.84 and 1,

Table 1.1   Failure time for the heart disease example.

Failure time (months)	1	1.5	2	3.2	4	4.3	5	6.1	7	7.3	8	8.1	8.5	9	10	10.5	11	12	15	16
Type of failure	MI	MI	D	MI	D	D	D	MI	D	MI	MI	D	D	D	MI	MI	MI	D	MI	D

resulting in a sum of 1.84 which, as a probability, is nonsensical since it is larger than 1. Hence, in the competing risks framework, in contrast to the cumulative incidence approach, $1 - KM$ cannot be interpreted as the probability of an event happening by time t.

1.4   TESTING IN THE COMPETING RISK FRAMEWORK

In the previous section it was shown that the classical (Kaplan–Meier) technique for summarizing time-to-event data is not recommended in the presence of competing risks. In contrast, when testing a covariate, the standard methods as well as the newly developed methods can be applied. The log-rank test and Cox regression are well established methods of analysis in the survival literature. These methods ignore the competing risks and test the 'pure' effect, which may be useful. In contrast, the more recent techniques developed by Pepe and Mori (1993), Gray (1988) and Fine and Gray (1999) take into account the competing risks. Therefore, the analysis of time-to-event data in the presence of competing risks has two main approaches: testing the 'pure' effect by ignoring the competing risks and incorporating the competing risks. Each of these methods gives a different clue regarding the effect of the covariate.

Choosing which test to use should be a collaborative effort between researcher and statistician. The statistician needs to understand the experiment and the researcher needs to understand the implications of using any of these methods. To illustrate the principles involved, a real-life example follows.

Hodgkin's disease (HD) is a type of cancer which is common among young people (the median age is 30 years). Let us consider a group of 616 patients diagnosed with early stage Hodgkin's disease, treated with radiation therapy. This is a subset of the dataset presented in Section 1.6.5. Since the early stage disease (stages I and II) is well controlled by treatment and the patients are young (80% of them younger than 45 years), they tend to live a long time after the treatment. Analysing this group of patients can give information about the late effects of radiation. Suppose that the event of interest is the incidence of second malignancy. Inevitably, some patients die before the appearance of another malignancy. Death without malignancy constitutes the competing risk. There are 84 patients for which a second malignancy was documented and 195 who died without a second malignancy. The remaining individuals did not experience any event and are considered censored. The main question is whether the younger group (aged 30 or younger) differs with respect to the occurrence of second malignancy compared to the older group (aged over 30). Since a malignancy is more likely to occur as one grows older, it is expected that the older group has more second malignancies than the younger one. Figure 1.2 shows the cumulative incidence curves for the second malignancy in the two groups and the *p*-values for

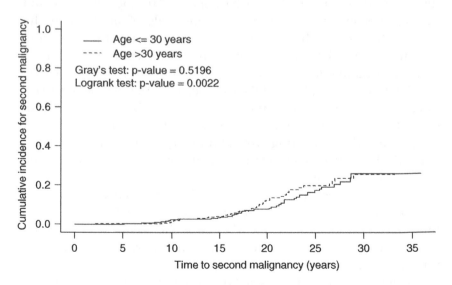

Figure 1.2 Cumulative incidence for malignancy by age group.

Gray's test and for the log-rank test. Counter-intuitively, Gray's test and the curves suggest that the two groups are similar. The log-rank test, which ignores the competing risks, seems to be more consistent with our prior expectations. The results of these tests are strikingly different because they convey different information. The cumulative incidence curves for the competing risk (death without second malignancy) in the two groups differ greatly (Figure 1.3). The older group has a far larger incidence of death without malignancy than the younger group.

It is to be expected that the older a person gets, the more likely he/she is to have other fatal conditions. Because an older person may die of other causes a second malignancy may not have a chance to be observed and therefore the two groups end up having a similar number of second malignancies, hence the non-significance of Gray's test. The log-rank test expresses the fact that if the deaths of other cases did not occur the probabilities for the second malignancy would be different in the two groups. A specific preventive measure for the second malignancy in the older population need not be taken since the

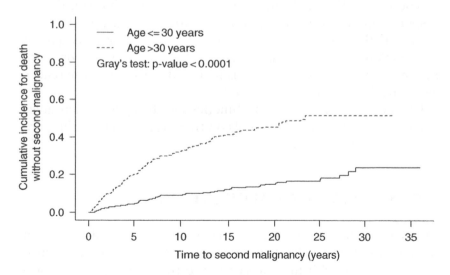

Figure 1.3 Cumulative incidence for death without second malignancy (competing risk).

number of malignancies is about the same as in the younger population. However, the significance of the log-rank test suggests that the biology of getting a second malignancy in the older population is different than in the younger group. Therefore, it may be worthwhile to analyse genetically the tumour tissue from the second malignancy and contrast the findings between the young and old population. In conclusion, the older patients do indeed have a higher risk of getting the second malignancy, but they also have a higher risk of getting other life-threatening diseases which makes the number of second malignancies observed about the same as in the younger group.

Suppose that this group of HD patients is compared with a group of patients registered at a hospital for a disease other than cancer who were not treated with radiation. In this case the log-rank test tells us whether the HD patients treated with radiation have a larger risk of second malignancy. One hypothesis which can be generated is that radiation causes second malignancies. Gray's test answers the question whether more second malignancies are observed in one group, a result which is sensitive to the group to which we compare the HD patients. Thus, Gray's test will give different results when the HD population is compared with a group of young, healthy individuals who came into the hospital due to a sports injury and with a group of young heart disease patients. However, the test takes into account the competing risks, giving information on the observed difference between groups. For more information on the interpretations included in this book the reader can consult Sections 3.3.3 and 4.1.

In conclusion, while both techniques can be applied each gives different information. More details on these tests and modelling are given in Chapters 5 and 6.

1.5   SAMPLE SIZE CALCULATION

One step in the process of planning a study is the calculation of the total number of subjects necessary to detect a specific difference in the outcome with the two types of error (α and β) set to pre-specified values. This section is intended for those researchers who do not wish to make these calculations themselves but employ a statistician for this purpose. Therefore, the focus is on conveying the general ideas involved and the necessary data that the researcher needs to supply to the statistician.

The sample size calculation in time-to-event analysis is more complex than for other types of endpoint. If the endpoint of a study is the average of some variable one only needs to know the difference to be detected, the standard deviation and, of course, the two types of error. To be able to calculate a sample size when the endpoint is a proportion, one only needs the two hypothesized proportions and the two types of error.

In survival analysis the necessary number of events is calculated first, followed by the total number of patients that produces the number of events needed. This is why more information is needed for the calculation of the sample size for time-to-event outcomes than for any other types of outcome. If the outcome is survival then besides the hypothesized percentage survival at a certain point in time one also needs to know the rate of accrual and the length of follow-up after the accrual ends. While the former helps to estimate the number of events necessary, the latter is used to calculate the number of individuals necessary to produce the required number of events. In addition, when competing risks are present, an estimate of the incidence of competing risks is needed. Extra care has to be given to the method used to estimate the hypothesized percentages for the event of interest as well as for the competing risks. Therefore, it is important to know whether the hypothesized percentages are based on the cumulative incidence approach or are obtained from an older study where $1 - KM$ was used. The computation of sample size is dealt with in Chapter 7.

1.6 EXAMPLES

This section presents the examples that will be used throughout this book. They are based on real-life examples for which relevant references are given where possible. However, the data are not identical to those used in the original publications. To eliminate missing data, some records have been excluded or changed. The missing values were substituted either by the median value, when there were very few (two or three), or by a randomly generated number from the same distribution as the original variable. Only a subset of the variables available in the original datasets are used in this book. The follow-up may not be the most recent or the same as that used in the published sources. Although we have modified the data, we have tried not to change them in a fundamental way. The types of events, their pattern of occurrence, and the way in which they were collected are the same as in the original studies. Time is calculated in years. These examples have been included to illustrate statistical issues that arise in practical research, and not for purposes of drawing medical conclusions. For each of the five real-life examples a portion of the data (20 records) is shown in tables together with a description of the variables. All these datasets can be downloaded from the website address given in the Preface and read in R or SAS (see Sections B.1.5 and B.2 in Appendix B).

1.6.1   Tamoxifen trial

In December 1992 a multicentre randomized clinical trial for patients with node negative breast cancer began accruing subjects. Between 1992 and 2000, a total of 769 women were randomized: 383 in the tamoxifen-alone arm (Tam) and 386 in the combined radiation and tamoxifen arm (RT+Tam). The last follow-up was conducted in the summer of 2002. Only those patients accrued at a single contributor institution are included here: 321 patients in the Tam arm and 320 in the RT+Tam arm. The original design was for an equivalence study with disease-free survival as the main endpoint. However, for the purpose of this book this fact will be ignored the data analysed as an effectiveness trial, investigating whether RT+Tam is better than Tam alone. The events recorded were local relapse, axillary relapse, distant relapse, second malignancy of any type, and death. The time of the first occurrence of each type, of event was documented. For example, if a patient experienced local relapse at 1 year, another local relapse at 2 years and an axillary relapse at 3 years, the only events recorded are the local relapse at 1 year and the axillary relapse at 3 years. The local relapse at 2 years is the second relapse of the same type and is not recorded. For each type of event there is a censoring variable, which indicates whether the event occurred.

The time was calculated in years from the date of randomization to occurrence of the event or last follow-up date. Table 1.2a contains a portion of the data and Table 1.2b contains the list of variables and their description. The clinical aspects of the study and details of the original analysis can be found elsewhere (Fyles *et al.*, 2004).

1.6.2   Hypoxia study

Between 1994 and 2000, 109 patients diagnosed with primary cervical cancer were treated at a cancer centre, and data on these patients were collected prospectively. Two tumour markers were investigated in this study: a hypoxia marker (HP5) and the interstitial fluid pressure (IFP). The oxygenation level, recorded in millimetres of mercury (mmHg), was measured in each tumour 25–30 times along a track, with 3–4 tracks per tumour. The hypoxia marker was defined as the percentage of measurements in a tumour that had oxygen level less than 5 mmHg. The IFP was measured at a number of locations in the tumour and a mean value per patient was calculated. More details on how HP5 and IFP were measured can be found in the original reports (Wong *et al.*, 1997; Milosevic *et al.*, 1998). The main goal of this study was to determine whether HP5 and IFP influence outcome, and if so, to point researchers toward new treatment strategies designed to target cells with low levels of oxygen or high levels of IFP. Full reports of the effect of IIP5 and IFP on outcome and a comprehensive description of the study can be found elsewhere (Fyles *et al.*, 2002; Milosevic *et al.*, 2001).

The outcome variables recorded for this study are response to treatment, relapse and death. Tables 1.3 contain a portion of the data and the description of the variables. The response to treatment is presented here in a simplified version: complete response (CR) when the tumour has completely disappeared after treatment and the patient was disease-free at the end of the treatment; and no response (NR) when either the tumour has not disappeared or the disease has progressed to other sites (see Figure 1.4). When the response is NR the location of disease is recorded in the appropriate fields: if disease progressed distantly then `disrec=Y`; if the tumour

Table 1.2a Tamoxifen trial: extract from the `tamrt` dataset.

stnum	tx	pathsize	hist	hrlevel	hgb	nodediss	age	survtime	stat	loctime	lcens	axltime	acens	distime	dcens	maltime	mcens
1	B	1	DUC	POS	140	Y	51	8.268	0	8.268	0	8.268	0	8.268	0	8.268	0
2	B	0.5	DUC	POS	138	Y	74	6.174	0	6.174	0	6.174	0	1.352	1	6.174	0
3	B	1.1	DUC	POS	157	Y	71	7.176	0	7.176	0	7.176	0	7.176	0	7.176	0
4	B	0.8	DUC	POS	136	Y	52	9.506	0	9.506	0	9.506	0	9.506	0	9.506	0
5	B	1.5	DUC	POS	123	Y	62	9.095	0	9.095	0	9.095	0	9.095	0	9.095	0
6	B	0.7	DUC	POS	122	Y	75	8.096	1	5.812	0	5.812	0	5.812	0	8.096	0
7	B	2.4	DUC	POS	139	Y	77	0.726	1	0.726	0	0.726	0	0.602	1	0.726	0
8	B	2	DUC	POS	142	Y	78	4.964	0	4.964	0	4.964	0	4.964	0	4.964	0
9	B	2	DUC	POS	121	Y	65	8.849	0	8.849	0	8.849	0	8.849	0	8.849	0
10	B	1.2	DUC	POS	132	Y	67	5.164	0	5.164	0	5.164	0	5.164	0	5.164	0
321	T	2.5	LOB	POS	134	Y	72	8.027	0	8.027	0	8.027	0	8.027	0	2.393	1
322	T	3	DUC	NEG	133	Y	70	3.242	1	0.925	1	3.242	0	3.242	0	2.281	1
323	T	0.8	DUC	POS	135	Y	66	9.284	0	9.284	0	9.284	0	9.284	0	9.284	0
324	T	1.2	DUC	POS	128	Y	56	9.700	0	9.700	0	9.700	0	9.700	0	9.700	0
325	T	0.4	DUC	POS	148	Y	57	9.676	0	9.676	0	9.676	0	9.676	0	9.676	0
326	T	2	DUC	POS	140	Y	56	9.624	0	4.747	1	9.624	0	9.624	0	9.624	0
327	T	1.1	DUC	NEG	152	Y	65	9.229	0	5.331	1	9.229	0	9.229	0	9.073	1
328	T	3	DUC	POS	154	Y	53	9.142	0	9.142	0	9.142	0	9.142	0	9.142	0
329	T	1	DUC	POS	141	Y	66	8.704	0	8.704	0	8.704	0	6.138	1	8.704	0
330	T	1	DUC	POS	136	Y	74	4.871	1	4.871	0	4.871	0	4.871	0	4.871	0

Table 1.2b Tamoxifen trial: description of variables in the dataset.

Variable name	Description
stnum	Patient ID
tx	Randomized treatment: T=tamoxifen, B=radiation + tamoxifen
Variables assessed at the time of randomization	
pathsize	Size of the tumour (cm)
hist	Histology: DUC=Ductal, LOB=Lobular, MED=Medullary, MIX=Mixed, OTH=Other
hrlevel	Hormone receptor level: NEG=Negative, POS=Positive
hgb	Haemoglobin (g/l)
nodediss	Whether axillary node dissection was done: Y=Yes, N=No
age	Age (years)
Outcome variables	
survtime	Time from randomization to death or last follow-up
stat	Status at last follow-up: 1=Dead, 0=Alive
loctime	Time from randomization to local relapse or last follow-up
lcens	Local relapse: 1=Yes, 0=No
axltime	Time from randomization to axillary relapse or last follow-up
acens	Axillary relapse: 1=Yes, 0=No
distime	Time from randomization to distant relapse or last follow-up
dcens	Distant relapse: 1=Yes, 0=No
maltime	Time from randomization to any second malignancy or last follow-up
mcens	Malignancy: 1=Yes, 0=No

did not disappear then `pelrec=Y`. If the patient had a complete response (CR) after treatment the disease may have relapsed either in the pelvis (`pelrec=Y`) or distantly (`disrec=Y`). Therefore, when `pelrec=Y` it may mean either that the patient did not respond to treatment or that the disease relapsed in the pelvis. The response to treatment indicates which of these cases applies. Note that for this dataset no death occurred before a relapse, thus death does not appear as an event. The time to event is calculated in years

Table 1.3a Hypoxia study: extract from the hypox dataset.

stnum	age	hgb	tumsize	IFP	HP5	resp	pelvicln	pelrec	disrec	survtime	stat	dftime	dfcens
1	78	119	7	8.0	32.14	CR	N	N	N	6.152	0	6.152	0
2	69	131	2	8.2	2.17	CR	N	N	N	8.008	0	8.008	0
3	55	126	10	8.6	52.33	NR	N	Y	N	0.621	1	0.003	1
4	55	141	8	3.3	3.26	CR	N	Y	Y	1.120	1	1.073	1
5	50	95	8	8.0	85.43	NR	Y	Y	N	1.292	1	0.003	1
6	57	132	8	20.0	19.35	CR	N	N	N	7.929	0	7.929	0
7	53	127	4	21.8	44.58	CR	E	N	N	8.454	0	8.454	0
8	62	142	5	31.6	59.68	CR	N	Y	Y	7.116	0	7.107	1
9	23	145	5	16.5	29.17	CR	N	N	N	8.378	0	8.378	0
10	57	142	3	31.5	85.71	CR	N	N	N	8.178	0	8.178	0
11	74	124	4	8.0	8.065	CR	N	N	N	3.395	1	3.395	1
12	67	133	5	12.8	77.63	NR	Y	Y	Y	1.016	1	0.003	1
13	72	133	4	18.4	33.33	CR	N	N	N	3.699	1	1.350	1
14	66	116	8	8.0	99.22	NR	E	Y	Y	0.630	1	0.003	1
15	47	82	10	21.0	66.29	CR	Y	N	Y	8.194	0	0.512	1
16	61	118	5	23.6	55.00	CR	N	N	Y	4.764	1	1.714	1
17	78	95	7	21.0	81.60	NR	N	Y	N	2.590	1	0.003	1
18	52	150	6	11.1	56.76	CR	N	N	N	7.707	0	7.707	0
19	33	119	7	14.6	52.04	CR	N	Y	Y	1.478	1	0.939	1
20	45	125	5	30.9	46.77	CR	N	N	N	7.316	0	7.316	0

Table 1.3b Hypoxia study: description of variables in the dataset.

Variable Name	Description
stnum	Patient ID

Variables assessed at the time of diagnosis

age	Age (years)
hgb	Haemoglobin (g/l)
tumsize	Tumour size (cm)
IFP	Interstitial fluid pressure (marker, mmHg)
HP5	Hypoxia marker (percentage of measurements less than 5 mmHg)
pelvicln	Pelvic node involvement: N=Negative, E=Equivocal, Y=Positive

Outcome variables

resp	Response after treatment: CR=Complete response, NR=No response
pelrec	Pelvic disease observed: Y=Yes, N=No
disrec	Distant disease observed: Y=Yes, N=No
survtime	Time from diagnosis to death or last follow-up time
stat	Status at last follow-up: 0=Alive, 1=Dead
dftime	Time from diagnosis to first failure (no response to treatment, relapse or death) or last follow-up
dfcens	Censoring variable: 1=Failure, 0=Censored

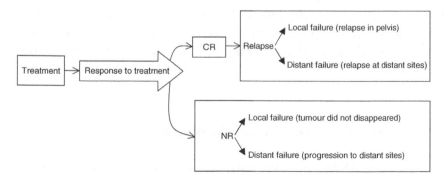

Figure 1.4 Types of failure in the hypoxia study.

from the date of diagnosis to first failure. Note that if the patient did not respond to treatment she was never disease-free. Therefore, the time to first failure is taken to be 1 day. For patients without any event the time is calculated up to the last follow-up date.

1.6.3   Follicular cell lymphoma study

A hospital database of lymphoma patient data was created at the Princess Margaret Hospital, Toronto, with records dating from 1967. Currently, the database is prospective, patients being entered as they register for treatment at the hospital. The subset of 541 patients that will be used throughout this book includes all patients identified as having follicular type lymphoma, registered for treatment at the hospital between 1967 and 1996, with early stage disease (I or II) and treated with radiation alone (RT) or with radiation and chemotherapy (CMT). The goal of this study was to report the long-term outcome in this group of patients. The outcome recorded included response to treatment, first relapse (local, distant or both) and death. The response to treatment is given here in a simplified version: CR is complete response and NR is no response. Those with a CR may have relapsed later locally, distantly, or both locally and distantly. Those with NR were never disease-free and are considered local failures. The time to first failure is calculated in years from the date of diagnosis. For the patients with no response the time to first failure is taken to be 1 day. For those with CR but without relapse, the time to first failure is calculated up to the last follow-up date. Part of the dataset and the list of variables are shown in Tables 1.4. A report on a part of this dataset can be found in Petersen *et al.* (2004b).

1.6.4   Bone marrow transplant study

In January 1996, a multicentre randomized clinical trial was initiated for patients with a myeloid malignancy who were to undergo an allogeneic bone marrow transplant. The donors in all cases were matched siblings. Traditionally, donated cells have been

Table 1.4a Follicular cell lymphoma study: extract from the `follic` dataset.

stnum	age	hgb	clinstg	ch	rt	resp	relsite	survtime	stat	dftime	dfcens
1	56	140	2		Y	CR	B	0.698	1	0.238	1
2	36	130	2		Y	CR	D	14.502	1	12.419	1
3	39	140	2	Y	Y	NR		4.914	1	0.003	1
4	37	140	1		Y	CR		15.685	1	15.685	1
5	61	110	2		Y	NR		0.235	1	0.003	1
6	69	120	1		Y	CR		8.419	1	8.419	1
7	57	110	2		Y	CR		25.150	1	25.150	1
8	32	120	2		Y	CR		31.102	0	31.102	0
9	24	110	2		Y	CR		14.574	0	14.574	0
10	49	110	2		Y	CR	B	22.664	1	0.808	1
11	44	130	2		Y	CR	D	15.261	1	5.615	1
12	82	120	1		Y	NR		1.725	1	0.003	1
13	58	130	1		Y	CR	D	15.559	1	13.049	1
14	32	140	2		Y	CR	D	2.563	1	0.151	1
15	51	140	2		Y	CR		29.667	1	29.667	1
16	73	130	2		Y	CR	D	3.305	1	2.193	1
17	64	130	1		Y	CR	D	1.999	1	0.405	1
18	56	129	1		Y	CR	D	11.614	1	11.184	1
19	38	160	2		Y	CR		11.274	0	11.274	0
20	68	160	2		Y	CR	D	4.736	1	4.005	1

Table 1.4b Follicular cell lymphoma study: description of variables in the dataset.

Variable name	Description
stnum	Patient ID

Variables assessed at the time of diagnosis

age	Age (years)
hgb	Haemoglobin (g/l)
clinstg	Clinical stage: 1=stage I, 2=stage II
ch	Chemotherapy: Y=Yes, blank=No
rt	Radiotherapy: Y=Yes, blank=No

Outcome variables

resp	Response after treatment: CR=Complete response, NR=No response
relsite	Site of relapse: L=Local, D=Distant, B=Local and Distant, blank=No relapse
survtime	Time from diagnosis to death or last follow-up
stat	Status: 1=Dead, 0=Alive
dftime	Time from diagnosis to first failure (no response, relapse or death) or last follow-up
dfcens	Censoring variable:1=Failure, 0=Censored

harvested from the pelvic bone of the donor (BM). This study was aimed at comparing the traditional method with a newer technique in which cells are collected from the peripheral blood of the donor (PB). These two cell collection methods formed the two arms of this study. The endpoint for which the study was designed was time to neutrophil recovery. In this book other types of endpoint will be examined: time to relapse, time to chronic graft versus host disease (CGVHD) and time to death. Only the first event of each type was recorded. The time is calculated in years from the date of transplant to the date of each specific event. In the situation where the patient did not experience any event, the time is calculated to the last follow-up date. For each type of event there is a censoring variable indicating whether the event occurred. Between 1996 and 2000, when the study closed, there were 228 patients accrued. In this book only the subgroup of 100 patients treated at the Princess Margaret Hospital are included. Tables 1.5 give a part of the dataset and the list of variables. A full report on this study can be found in Couban *et al.* (2002).

1.6.5   Hodgkin's disease study

Patients treated for Hodgkin's disease at the Princess Margaret Hospital between 1968 and 1986 were entered into a database and their records were updated regularly. There are 865 records in this dataset. All patients have early stage disease (I or II) and were treated either with radiation (RT) or with radiation and chemotherapy (CMT). The goal of this study was to report the long-term outcome in this group of patients. The outcome recorded included the first relapse, the second malignancy (malignancy diagnosed after the Hodgkin's disease) and death. The time to failure is given in years and is calculated from the date of diagnosis. Part of the dataset and the list of variables are shown in Tables 1.6. A report on a part of this dataset can be found in Petersen *et al.* (2004a).

Table 1.5a Bone marrow transplant study: extract from the bmt dataset.

stnum	dx	tx	extent	age	survtime	reltime	agvhtime	cgvhtime	stat	rcens	agvhdgd	agvh	cgvh
1	CML	PB	L	36	4.895	4.895	0.099	0.520	0	0	1	1	1
2	AML	PB	L	57	3.474	0.753	0.101	0.408	1	1	3	1	1
3	CML	PB	L	48	4.950	4.950	4.950	0.348	0	0	0	0	1
4	AML	PB	L	52	4.643	4.643	0.057	0.482	0	0	2	1	1
5	AML	PB	L	45	4.066	4.066	0.137	0.378	0	0	3	1	1
6	AML	PB	L	47	1.558	0.416	0.055	1.558	1	1	3	1	0
7	CML	PB	L	40	4.512	4.512	0.09	0.381	0	0	1	1	1
8	AML	PB	L	38	4.041	4.041	0.082	0.914	0	0	3	1	1
9	AML	PB	L	41	4.164	4.164	0.055	0.923	0	0	2	1	1
10	CML	PB	L	50	4.011	4.011	4.011	0.397	0	0	0	0	1
50	CML	BM	L	45	4.572	4.572	0.066	0.619	0	0	3	1	1
51	AML	BM	L	45	4.616	4.616	0.101	0.452	0	0	3	1	1
52	AML	BM	L	42	4.000	4.000	0.027	0.290	0	0	2	1	1
53	CML	BM	L	22	4.238	4.238	4.238	0.479	0	0	0	0	1
54	AML	BM	L	47	0.110	0.110	0.074	0.110	1	0	4	1	0
55	AML	BM	L	48	4.030	4.030	0.101	0.857	0	0	2	1	1
56	AML	BM	L	49	3.124	2.527	0.115	1.993	1	1	2	1	1
57	CML	BM	L	38	0.515	0.515	0.079	0.463	1	0	2	1	1
58	CML	BM	L	39	4.222	3.149	0.085	0.496	0	1	1	1	1
59	CML	BM	L	40	4.027	4.027	0.104	0.422	0	0	3	1	1

Table 1.5b   Bone marrow transplant study: description of variables in the dataset.

Variable name	Description
stnum	Patient ID
Variables assessed at the time of randomization	
tx	Randomized treatment:
	BM=cells harvested from the bone marrow,
	PB=cell harvested from the peripheral blood
dx	Diagnosis:
	AML=acute myeloid leukaemia,
	CML=chronic myeloid leukaemia
	MDS=myelodysplastic syndrome
extent	Extent of disease: L=limited, E=extensive
age	Age (years)
Outcome variables	
survtime	Time from date of transplant to death or last follow-up
reltime	Time from date of transplant to relapse or last follow-up
agvhtime	Time from date of transplant to acute GVHD or last follow-up
cgvhtime	Time from date of transplant to chronic GVHD or last follow-up
stat	Status: 1=Dead, 0=Alive
rcens	Relapse: 1=Yes, 0=No
agvhdgd	Grade of acute GVHD
agvh	Acute GVHD: 1=Yes, 0=No
cgvh	Chronic GVHD: 1=Yes, 0=No

Table 1.6a Hodgkin's disease study: extract from the hd dataset.

stnum	age	sex	trtgiven	medwidsi	extranod	clinstg	survtime	stat	dftime	dfcens	rcens	cscens	maltime	mcens
1	64	F	RT	N	N	1	3.102	1	3.102	1	0	0	3.102	0
2	63	M	RT	N	N	1	15.885	1	15.885	1	0	0	15.885	0
3	17	M	RT	N	N	2	1.103	1	0.882	1	1	1	1.103	0
4	63	M	RT	N	N	2	13.120	0	13.120	1	0	0	13.120	0
5	21	M	RT	L	N	2	35.923	0	35.923	0	0	0	35.923	0
6	37	M	RT	N	N	1	1.834	1	1.106	1	1	1	1.834	0
7	41	M	RT	N	N	2	2.494	1	2.494	1	1	1	2.494	0
8	35	M	RT	N	N	2	7.767	1	0.003	1	1	1	7.767	0
9	27	F	CMT	N	N	2	28.841	0	4.052	1	1	0	25.06	1
10	32	M	RT	N	N	2	28.093	0	28.093	0	0	0	28.093	0
11	68	F	RT	N	N	1	1.706	1	1.689	1	1	1	1.706	0
12	27	F	RT	N	N	2	18.33	1	1.210	1	1	0	18.33	0
13	61	M	RT	N	N	1	1.051	1	1.051	1	1	1	1.051	0
14	27	M	RT	S	N	2	1.303	1	0.537	1	1	1	1.303	0
15	34	M	RT	N	N	2	2.689	1	0.715	1	1	1	2.689	0
16	26	M	RT	N	N	1	2.185	1	1.101	1	1	1	2.185	0
17	19	M	RT	L	N	2	5.520	1	1.634	1	1	1	5.520	0
18	19	M	RT	N	N	2	0.671	1	0.660	1	1	1	0.671	0
19	31	M	RT	N	N	2	32.271	0	32.271	0	0	0	32.271	0
20	17	M	RT	N	N	1	30.467	0	30.467	0	0	0	30.467	0

Table 1.6b Hodgkin's disease study: description of variables in the dataset.

Variable name	Description
stnum	Patient ID
Variables assessed at the time of diagnosis	
age	Age (years)
sex	Haemoglobin (g/l)
trtgiven	Radiotherapy: RT= Radiation, CMT=Chemotherapy and radiation
medwidsi	Size of mediastinum involvement: N= No, S= Small, L= Large
extranod	Extranodal disease: Y=Extranodal disease, N= Nodal disease
clinstg	Clinical stage: 1=Stage I, 2=Stage II
Outcome variables	
survtime	Time from diagnosis to death or last follow-up
stat	Status: 0=Alive, 1=Dead
dftime	Time from diagnosis to first failure (relapse or death) or last follow-up
dfcens	Censoring variable:0=Censored, 1=Failure
rcens	Response and relapse: 0= Disease-free, 1= Relapse or no response to treatment
cscens	Cause specific death: 0= Death due to other causes or alive, 1= Death due to Hodgkin's disease
maltime	Time from diagnosis of Hodgkin's disease to second malignancy or last follow-up
mcens	Second malignancy: 0= No, 1= Yes

2

Survival – basic concepts

2.1 INTRODUCTION

The analysis of competing risks data requires a basic understanding of the statistical methods used for censored survival data. This chapter presents a brief review of those methods that will be referred to later in the text. Readers familiar with survival analysis may choose to skip this chapter.

2.2 DEFINITIONS AND BACKGROUND FORMULAE

2.2.1 Introduction

There are many instances in clinical research practice where the time to a particular event is of interest. For example, in the study of an in-patient population, the time from admission to hospital until the patient is discharged might be of interest. Similarly, a clinical trial comparing two chemotherapy regimes for colon cancer might have the time between diagnosis and first recurrence as the primary outcome measure.

The nature of these time-to-event or lifetime data requires the use of special statistical techniques. Typically, the exact time to

---

Competing Risks: A Practical Perspective   M. Pintilie
© 2006 John Wiley & Sons, Ltd

the event is observed for only a fraction of the patients included
in the study. For all others, what is known is that the time to
the event is greater than the follow-up available. This is known as
censoring. Suppose, for instance, that a patient is followed for 5 years
subsequent to chemotherapy for colon cancer and does not have a
recurrence during that time period. Although the time to recurrence
remains unknown, this patient provides valuable information about
the probability of remaining free of recurrence for at least 5 years.
Survival analysis methods make use of all observations, including
those for which an event is not yet recorded. Censoring is discussed
further in Section 2.2.4.

2.2.2   Basic mathematical formulae

Often the goal of studies that collect time-to-event data is to estimate
the probability that the event occurs after a given point in time.
As an example, it might be of interest to estimate the probability
that the symptom-free time between bronchitic episodes is at least
1 month in a population of chronic bronchitis patients. The time
to event can be continuous or discrete. Although in this book the
discrete situation is mostly of interest, this section gives the formulae
for both cases. In addition to the usual functions given in statistics –
the cumulative distribution function (cdf) and probability density
function (pdf), those concepts specific to survival analysis – the
survivor function and hazard function – are presented.

Continuous distributions

Let T denote the random variable for the time to event, considered
as continuous. The *survivor function* is defined as the probability
that the time to event exceeds some specified time t:

$$S(t) = P(T > t). \tag{2.1}$$

If $F(t)$ is the cdf of the time to event, then the survivor function
can be expressed in terms of the cdf, and vice versa:

$$S(t) = P(T > t) = 1 - P(T \leq t) = 1 - F(t).$$

The pdf, $f(t)$, can be found from either the survivor function or the cdf by differentiating:

$$f(t) = \frac{dF(t)}{dt} = \frac{d\{1 - S(t)\}}{dt} = -\frac{dS(t)}{dt}.$$

Alternatively, if the density function is known, both the cdf and the survivor function can be found by integrating the pdf. The cdf is $F(t) = \int_0^t f(x)dx$ and, similarly, the survivor function is $S(t) = \int_t^\infty f(x)dx$.

The *hazard function* is the instantaneous event rate for an individual who has made it to time t without experiencing the event. When the event of interest is death, this is the instantaneous death rate for an individual who has survived to time t. This function is often of interest in the analysis of time-to-event data because it illustrates how the instantaneous event rate varies over time. Mathematically, the hazard function is the conditional probability of an event occurring within a narrow window of time, say between t and $t + \delta t$, given that there was no event up to time t. Since δt is very small, the limit of the conditional probability when $\delta t \to 0$ is calculated. Therefore, the hazard function is defined as:

$$h(t) = \lim_{\delta t \to 0} \left\{ \frac{P(t < T \le t + \delta t | T > t)}{\delta t} \right\}. \tag{2.2}$$

This expression can be algebraically modified to obtain a more palatable form:

$$
\begin{aligned}
h(t) &= \lim_{\delta t \to 0} \left\{ \frac{P(t < T \le t + \delta t)}{\delta t P(T > t)} \right\} \\
&= \lim_{\delta t \to 0} \left\{ \frac{F(t + \delta t) - F(t)}{\delta t P(T > t)} \right\} \\
&= \frac{f(t)}{S(t)}.
\end{aligned}
\tag{2.3}
$$

The survivor function can be expressed in terms of the hazard function by noticing that

$$h(t) = -\frac{d}{dt} \{ \log S(t) \},$$

which when integrated becomes $\log S(t) = -\int_0^t h(x)dx$, and it follows that

$$S(t) = \exp\left\{-\int_0^t h(x)dx\right\}.$$

The *cumulative hazard function* is defined as $H(t) = \int_0^t h(x)dx$. Therefore, the survivor function can also be written as

$$S(t) = \exp\{-H(t)\}.$$

The relationships between these various functions used in the analysis of time-to-event data are summarized in Table 2.1.

Discrete distributions

Similar formulae can be derived for the case when the time-to-event random variable, T, has a discrete distribution. Suppose that T can take on the values $t_1, t_2, t_3, \ldots$ where $0 \le t_1 < t_2 < \ldots$ and its probability function is $p(t_j) = P(T = t_j)$. As in the continuous case, the survivor function is defined as $S(t) = P(T > t)$. In this case, though, it is calculated as a sum rather than an integral:

$$S(t) = P(T > t) = \sum_{t_j > t} p(t_j). \tag{2.4}$$

The hazard function for discrete time-to-event random variables is defined as

$$h(t_j) = P(T = t_j | T > t_{j-1}) = \frac{p(t_j)}{S(t_{j-1})}, \qquad \text{for } j = 1, 2, \ldots.$$

Note that $P(T \ge t_j) = S(t_{j-1})$ and since $p(t_j) = S(t_{j-1}) - S(t_j)$ (from (2.4)), it follows that the hazard function can be written as $h(t_j) = 1 - S(t_j)/S(t_{j-1})$. Using this last relationship and induction, the survivor function can be written in terms of the hazard function as

$$S(t) = \prod_{t_j \le t} (1 - h(t_j)). \tag{2.5}$$

There is no uniform agreement on how best to define the cumulative hazard function for the discrete case. One definition, which is

Table 2.1 Basic mathematical formulae.

Function	Continuous distributions		Discrete distributions	
	Definition	Relationship to other functions	Definition	Relationship to other functions
Cumulative distribution	$F(t) = P(T \leq t)$	$F(t) = \int_0^t f(x)dx$	$F(t) = P(T \leq t)$	$F(t) = \sum_{t_j \leq t} p(t_j)$
Probability density	$f(t) = \dfrac{d}{dt}F(t)$	$f(t) = -\dfrac{d}{dt}S(t)$	$p(t_j) = P(T = t_j)$	$p(t_j) = S(t_{j-1}) - S(t_j)$
Survivor	$S(t) = P(T > t)$	$S(t) = 1 - F(t)$ $= \int_t^\infty f(x)dx$ $= \exp\{-H(t)\}$	$S(t) = P(T > t)^*$	$S(t) = 1 - F(t)$ $= \sum_{t_j > t} p(t_j)$ $= \exp\{-H_2(t)\}$
Hazard	$h(t) = \lim_{\delta t \to 0}\left\{\dfrac{P(t \leq T < t+\delta t \mid T > t)}{\delta t}\right\}$	$h(t) = f(t)/S(t)$ $= -\dfrac{d}{dt}\log S(t)$	$h(t_j) = P(T = t_j \mid T \geq t_j)$ $H_1(t) = \sum_{t_j \leq t} h(t_j)$	$h(t_j) = p(t_j)/S(t_{j-1})$
Cumulative hazard	$H(t) = \int_0^t h(x)dx$	$H(t) = -\log S(t)$	$H_2(t) = -\sum_{t_j \leq t}\log\{1 - h(t_j)\}$	$H_2(t) = -\log S(t)$

* Probability function

appealing because it is intuitively easy to understand, especially in applied settings, is

$$H_1(t) = \sum_{t_j \leq t} h(t_j).$$

This definition, however, does not preserve the property $S(t) = \exp\{-H_1(t)\}$ that was seen in the continuous case. An alternate definition that maintains this relationship is

$$H_2(t) = -\sum_{t_j \leq t} \log\left(1 - h(t_j)\right) = -\log S(t).$$

When the hazard at each time point is small, these two definitions yield similar results.

2.2.3 Common parametric distributions

Although in this book the focus is on nonparametric methods in the analysis of lifetime data, the application of parametric models can be very useful. In cases where the proposed distribution is appropriate, parametric inference will be more efficient than methods that assume no form for the distribution. Ignoring the form of the distribution, if known, can lead to lack of precision. Several distributions or families of distributions are often used in research to model time-to-event data. Frequently, the choice of a particular distribution is based on empirical evidence, where the model has been identified as describing the data well.

The exponential, Weibull and log-logistic distributions are easy to work with in the sense that there are simple mathematical expressions for the survivor and hazard functions. Other distributions, such as the gamma, generalized gamma and lognormal distributions, may seem at first glance somewhat forbidding as they require numerical methods to obtain the survivor function. Some distributions that are often found to describe continuous lifetime data well are presented in Table 2.2 for reference.

Table 2.2 Parametric models for time-to-event data.

Distribution	$f(t)$	$F(t)$	$S(t)$	$h(t)$	$H(t)$
Exponential	$\lambda e^{-\lambda t}$	$1 - e^{-\lambda t}$	$e^{-\lambda t}$	λ	λt
Weibull	$\lambda\theta t^{\theta-1}\exp\{-\lambda t^\theta\}$	$1-\exp\{-\lambda t^\theta\}$	$\exp\{-\lambda t^\theta\}$	$\lambda\theta t^{\theta-1}$	λt^θ
Gamma	$\lambda^\theta t^{\theta-1} e^{-\lambda t}$	$\Pi(\theta,\lambda t)^\dagger$	$1-\Pi(\theta,\lambda t)$	$f(t)/S(t)$	$-\log S(t)$
Generalized gamma	$\dfrac{\alpha\lambda^\theta t^{\alpha\theta-1}\exp\{-\lambda t^\alpha\}}{\Gamma(\theta)}$	$\Pi(\theta,\lambda t^\alpha)^\dagger$	$1-\Pi(\theta,\lambda t^\alpha)$	$f(t)/S(t)$	$-\log S(t)$
Lognormal	$\dfrac{\exp\left\{-\dfrac{1}{2}\left(\dfrac{\log t-\mu}{\sigma}\right)^2\right\}}{\sigma t\sqrt{2\pi}}$	$\Phi\left(\dfrac{\log t-\mu}{\sigma}\right)^\ddagger$	$1-\Phi\left(\dfrac{\log t-\mu}{\sigma}\right)$	$f(t)/S(t)$	$-\log S(t)$
Log-logistic	$\dfrac{\lambda\theta t^{\theta-1}}{(1+\lambda t^\theta)^2}$	$\dfrac{\lambda t^\theta}{1+\lambda t^\theta}$	$\dfrac{1}{1+\lambda t^\theta}$	$\dfrac{\lambda\theta t^{\theta-1}}{1+\lambda t^\theta}$	$\log(1+\lambda t^\theta)$

† Π is the incomplete gamma function: $\Pi(\theta,\lambda t)=\int_0^t \lambda^\theta t^{\theta-1}e^{-\lambda t}dt/\Gamma(\theta)$.
‡ Φ is the cdf of the standard normal distribution.

2.2.4 Censoring and assumptions

As was mentioned in Section 2.2.1, censoring occurs when the exact time to event is not observed for some individuals. For censored observations all that is known is the lower or upper bound of the time to event.

An observation is said to be *right censored* if it is known that the time to event is greater than or equal to some cut-off point, K. In other words, right censoring means that the event of interest does not occur during an observation period of length K. This is the case in many clinical trials with a fixed follow-up period of K years. It is also possible for observations to be *left censored*. In this case, the time to event is known to be less than or equal to some cut-off point, K. Left censoring is not as common as right censoring, and throughout the remainder of this text it will be assumed that all censored data have been right censored.

The manner in which data are collected determines the properties of the censoring mechanism. *Type II censoring* occurs if at the outset of the study it is decided to observe the exact times of the first r events. Alternatively, the design of the study can stipulate that the individuals are followed for a fixed period of time, K; this is *Type I censoring*.

A more complex version of Type I censoring arises when a decision has been made to cease observation on a fixed calendar date, such as 1 June 2008, regardless of when individuals were enrolled in a study. Suppose a clinical trial will accrue subjects between 1 January 2007 and 30 April 2007. Since it is known in advance that study follow-up will be stopped on 1 June 2008, the censoring time for each individual is known at the time of enrolment in the study and their censoring times are different. In subsequent chapters, it is assumed that this form of Type I censoring has been used.

The occurrence of other events can also lead to censoring, and this is especially true in a competing risks situation. In a study whose goal is to estimate time to death due to heart attack, death due to any other cause will result in censoring. For simplicity, suppose that all the other deaths are due to malignancy. The heart condition that leads to heart attack and the occurrence of a malignancy are both prevalent in the older population. Therefore, the censoring due to cancer death is not independent of the heart attack death. This is called *informative censoring*. In contrast, *non-informative censoring* happens when time to censoring and time to event are independent.

2.3   ESTIMATION AND HYPOTHESIS TESTING

2.3.1   Estimating the hazard and survivor functions

A commonly used method for describing time-to-event data is the product-limit estimate of the survivor function first proposed by Kaplan and Meier (1958). Recall that the survivor function specifies the probability that the time to event is greater than t. In the case where there is no censoring, the product-limit estimator is identical to the empirical estimate of the survivor function, which is obtained simply by calculating the proportion of individuals who have experienced the event by a certain time point, t. This approach needs to be modified when some observations are censored.

Suppose that $t_1, t_2, \ldots, t_r$ are the unique failure time points such that $t_1 < t_2 < \ldots < t_r$. Let d_j be the number of events that occur at time t_j, and n_j the number of individuals at risk of experiencing the event immediately prior to t_j. Then the product-limit estimator of the survivor function is:

$$\hat{S}(t) = \prod_{t_j \leq t} \left(\frac{n_j - d_j}{n_j} \right).$$

(2.6)

In Appendix A we give the maximum likelihood estimation of this expression. The variance of $\hat{S}(t)$ is estimated using Greenwood's formula:

$$\widehat{\mathrm{Var}} \left(\hat{S}(t) \right) = \left\{ \hat{S}(t) \right\}^2 \sum_{t_j \leq t} \frac{d_j}{n_j \left(n_j - d_j \right)}.$$

(2.7)

For large sample sizes $\hat{S}(t)$ has an approximately normal distribution. Therefore, a simple way to obtain the $100(1 - \alpha)\%$ confidence interval for $\hat{S}(t)$ is

$$\hat{S}(t) \pm z_{1-\alpha/2} \sqrt{\widehat{\mathrm{Var}} \left(\hat{S}(t) \right)},$$

(2.8)

where z_α is the α quantile of the standard normal distribution (e.g. if $\alpha = 0.05$, then $z_{1-\alpha/2} = 1.96$). However, this confidence interval may include negative values or values greater than 1. To avoid this difficulty, Kalbfleisch and Prentice (1980) propose the confidence interval

$$\left[\hat{S}(t)\right]^{\exp[\pm A]},$$ (2.9)

where

$$A = \frac{z_{1-\alpha/2}\sqrt{\widehat{\mathrm{Var}}\left(\hat{S}(t)\right)}}{\hat{S}(t)\log\left(\hat{S}(t)\right)}.$$

Some mathematical details regarding this expression can be found in Section A.2.

Note that the formulae given are for calculating the pointwise confidence interval – that is, at any time point, the probability that the survival is within the limits of the confidence interval is $1 - \alpha$. The confidence band is defined as the band within the limits of which the survival at any point in time lies with probability $1 - \alpha$. Hall and Wellner (1980) show how to calculate confidence bands for survival.

An estimate of the cumulative hazard function can be obtained from the product-limit estimate of the survivor function: $\hat{H}(t) = -\log\left\{\hat{S}(t)\right\}$. Alternatively, the cumulative hazard function can be estimated using a method proposed by Nelson (1972) and by Aalen (1978b),

$$\hat{H}(t) = \sum_{t_j \leq t} \frac{d_j}{n_j},$$ (2.10)

and is 0 prior to the time of the first uncensored event. For large sample sizes, the Nelson–Aalen estimator and the product-limit-based estimator are similar.

Another summary measure often reported in medical literature is the median survival, which is defined as the time at which the survival is 0.5. Note that when the survivor function does not reach this mark (the entire curve is above 0.5) then the median survival is not estimable.

2.3.2 Nonparametric testing: log-rank and Wilcoxon tests

It is often of interest to test hypotheses about the equality of two or more survivor functions. Two commonly used nonparametric procedures for conducting such tests are the log-rank test, also known as the Mantel–Haenszel test, and the Wilcoxon test.

First, we present the formulae for the comparison between two groups are presented first, followed by more general formulae for m groups. As before, the unique, ordered failure times for all records (regardless of the group) are denoted by $t_1 < t_2 < \ldots < t_r$. Let d_{1j} be the number of failures and n_{1j} the numbers at risk in group 1 at time t_j. Let d_{2j} and n_{2j} be the corresponding numbers for group 2. Then $d_j = d_{1j} + d_{2j}$ represents the number of failures in both groups at time t_j and $n_j = n_{1j} + n_{2j}$ is the numbers at risk in both groups at time t_j.

If the survival is the same in both groups then the expected number of failures for group 1 at t_j is $e_{1j} = n_{1j}\frac{d_j}{n_j}$. The test is based on the difference between the observed d_{1j} and the expected e_{1j} of the form

$$U = \sum_{j=1}^{r} \left(d_{1j} - n_{1j}\frac{d_j}{n_j} \right). \tag{2.11}$$

The variance can be estimated as

$$\widehat{\mathrm{Var}}(U) = \sum_{j=1}^{r} \frac{n_{1j}n_{2j}d_j(n_j - d_j)}{n_j^2(n_j - 1)}.$$

The log-rank test is then given by the statistic

$$S = \frac{U^2}{\widehat{\mathrm{Var}}(U)},$$

which is known to be χ^2 distributed with 1 degree of freedom.

The Wilcoxon test is a weighted sum of the differences between observed and expected numbers of failures using n_j as weight. The homologous formulae are:

$$U_W = \sum_{j=1}^{r} \left\{ n_j \left(d_{1j} - n_{1j} \frac{d_j}{n_j} \right) \right\}, \qquad (2.12)$$

$$\widehat{Var}(U_W) = \sum_{j=1}^{r} \frac{n_{1j} n_{2j} d_j (n_j - d_j)}{(n_j - 1)}$$

The Wilcoxon test is then

$$S_W = \frac{U_W^2}{\widehat{Var}(U_W)},$$

which is also χ^2 distributed with one degree of freedom.

By using the number of individuals at risk as a weight, the Wilcoxon test gives greater weight to the earlier part of the curve where the sample size is larger than to the later time points when only a few individuals remain at risk. Hence, when the intention is to capture the early differences between the survivor functions the Wilcoxon test is more discriminatory than the log-rank test. The log-rank test is more efficient when the hazards are proportional. This means that the ratio of the hazards between the compared groups is constant over time, or that the hazards change in the same way in all groups. Table 2.3 gives such an example. While

Table 2.3   Example illustrating the concept of proportional hazards.

Time	Hazard Group 1	Hazard Group 2	Hazard Group 3	Hazard ratio Group 1 : Group 2	Hazard ratio Group 1 : Group 3
1	0.1	0.05	0.2	2	0.5
2	0.2	0.1	0.4	2	0.5
3	0.2	0.1	0.4	2	0.5
4	0.3	0.15	0.6	2	0.5
5	0.2	0.1	0.4	2	0.5
6	0.1	0.05	0.2	2	0.5
7	0.05	0.025	0.1	2	0.5

the hazard changes over time for each group, the ratio between group 1 and group 2 is always constant (=2) and between group 1 and group 3 is 0.5.

Note that U is written in terms of group 1 and that

$$U \text{ (group 1)} + U \text{ (group 2)} = 0,$$

$$\text{Var} \left(U \text{ (group 1)} \right) = \text{Var} \left(U \text{ (group 2)} \right).$$

It follows that the test statistics, as expected, do not depend whether they are written in terms of group 1 or group 2.

In the general case, for m groups, the log-rank test statistics has the quadratic form

$$\mathbf{U} \mathbf{\Sigma}^{-1} \mathbf{U}^t \qquad (2.13)$$

where $\mathbf{U}$ is a vector of length $m-1$ where each term is similar to ((2.11)), $\mathbf{U}^t$ is the transpose of the vector $\mathbf{U}$ and $\mathbf{\Sigma}$ is the variance–covariance matrix of size $m-1$. In particular, the elements of $\mathbf{U}$ are

$$u_k = \sum_{j=1}^{r} \left(d_{kj} - n_{kj} \frac{d_j}{n_j} \right), \qquad k = 1, 2, \ldots, m-1,$$

and the elements of $\mathbf{\Sigma}$ are

$$\sigma_{kk'} = \sum_{j=1}^{r} \frac{n_{kj} d_j (n_j - d_j)}{n_j (n_j - 1)} \left(\delta_{kk'} - \frac{n_{k'j}}{n_j} \right), \qquad k, k' = 1, 2, \ldots, m-1$$

Where

$$\delta_{kk'} = \begin{cases} 1, & \text{if } k = k', \\ 0, & \text{if } k \neq k'. \end{cases}$$

Under the null hypothesis the statistic in (2.13) has a χ^2 distribution with $m-1$ degrees of freedom.

The general Wilcoxon test for m groups has a similar form:

$$\mathbf{U}_W \mathbf{\Sigma}_W^{-1} \mathbf{U}_W^t \qquad (2.14)$$

with the elements of $\mathbf{U}_W$ given by

$$u_k = \sum_{j=1}^{r} \left\{ n_j \left(d_{kj} - n_{kj} \frac{d_j}{n_j} \right) \right\}, \qquad k = 1, 2, \ldots, m-1,$$

and the elements of the variance–covariance matrix

$$\sigma_{kk'} = \sum_{j=1}^{r} \frac{n_j n_{kj} d_j \left(n_j - d_j\right)}{\left(n_j - 1\right)} \left(\delta_{kk'} - \frac{n_{k'j}}{n_j}\right), \quad k, k' = 1, 2, \ldots, m-1$$

where

$$\delta_{kk'} = \begin{cases} 1, & \text{if } k = k', \\ 0, & \text{if } k \neq k'. \end{cases}$$

2.3.3   Proportional hazards model

This section presents the theoretical background for building a model under the assumption of proportional hazards. The hazard for an individual i with a given set of covariates $x_{1i}, x_{2i}, \ldots, x_{mi}$ can be decomposed into two parts: one that involves time but not the covariates, and one that involves the covariates but not time. Hence,

$$h_i(t) = \exp\{\beta_1 x_{1i} + \ldots + \beta_m x_{mi}\} h_0(t), \qquad (2.15)$$

where $h_0(t)$ is the baseline hazard function and $\beta_1, \beta_2, \ldots, \beta_m$ are the parameters or the coefficients which need to be estimated. As before, $t_1 < t_2 < \ldots < t_r$ are the unique, ordered failure time points. When there are no ties the estimates for the coefficients $\beta_1, \beta_2, \ldots, \beta_m$ are obtained by maximizing the partial likelihood (Cox, 1972)

$$L(\beta_1, \beta_2, \ldots, \beta_m) = \prod_{j=1}^{r} \left(\frac{\exp\{\beta_1 x_{1j} + \ldots + \beta_m x_{mj}\}}{\sum_{i \in R_j} \exp\{\beta_1 x_{1i} + \ldots + \beta_m x_{mi}\}} \right), \quad (2.16)$$

where the product is taken over all failure times t_j and R_j represents the set of individuals still at risk at t_j. The maximization of the partial likelihood is obtained through an iterative process best done on computer and the estimates $\hat{\beta}_1, \hat{\beta}_2, \ldots, \hat{\beta}_m$ do not have a closed form. Breslow (1974) and Efron (1977) suggested ways to handle tied observations. Easy-to-follow descriptions of these methods can be found in Collett (2003) and Therneau and

Grambsch (2000). The confidence interval for each coefficient $\hat{\beta}_k$, $k = 1, 2, \ldots, m$, is constructed as usual, $\hat{\beta}_k \pm z_{1-\alpha/2} \hat{\sigma}_{\beta_k}$, where z_α is the α quantile of the standard normal distribution. The Wald test of the hypothesis $H_0 : \beta_k = 0$ versus the alternative $H_a : \beta_k \neq 0$ is the test statistic $\hat{\beta}_k / \hat{\sigma}_{\beta_k}$ which follows the standard normal distribution.

2.4 SOFTWARE FOR SURVIVAL ANALYSIS

Currently, there are many statistical programs available. In this book the examples are analysed using SAS and R – the former because it is widely applied, and the latter because it has a package that deals with competing risks. Appendix B gives some details about R. Suffice it to say here that R has a very similar syntax to S-PLUS and many functions are available in both programs. There is a wealth of information on how to use SAS procedures. Specifically for survival analysis, besides the SAS manuals one can consult Allison (1995) and Cantor (2003). Since R and S-PLUS are so similar one could use the S-PLUS documentation. The book written by Therneau and Grambsch (2000) gives an excellent description of the use of functions specific to survival analysis in S-PLUS.

It is assumed that the reader has some experience of using these programs, and the complete syntax and examples are not given. A complete coverage of this topic would extend over much more than one chapter. The intention is to remind the reader of these procedures and functions.

The main procedures for nonparametric or semiparametric survival analysis in SAS are `proc lifetest` and `proc phreg`. The former outputs the product-limit estimator of the survivor function for each of the m groups and prints the results of both the log-rank and Wilcoxon test. The latter builds the Cox proportional hazards model.

In R the `survfit` function in combination with the `summary` function estimates the survivor function. The function `survdiff` performs the log-rank and Wilcoxon tests and `coxph` builds the Cox proportional hazards model.

2.5 CLOSING REMARKS

This chapter has given a brief overview of statistical methods for time-to-event data when there are no competing risks. Methods for competing risks build on these techniques. The survivor and hazard functions for both continuous and discrete time-to-event variables were introduced. The nonparametric log-rank and Wilcoxon methods for testing for differences between two or more survivor functions were presented as well as the basis for the Cox proportional hazards model. The log-rank and Wilcoxon tests are special cases of a more general class of rank tests, the details of which are not included here. There are many books on survival which can be consulted. Lawless (1982), Kalbfleisch and Prentice (2002) give a good theoretical background. Others (Marubini and Valsecchi, 1995; Collett, 2003) are more practical in nature. The use of SAS and R when analysing survival data in the absence of competing risks is beyond the scope of this book, and no details or examples are given.

3

Competing risks –
definitions

3.1 RECOGNIZING COMPETING RISKS

3.1.1 Practical approaches

The situation in which competing risks are present has been expressed in different ways by different authors. Since many of these descriptions shed light on different aspects of the competing risks situation, several are presented here in order to best illustrate the point. Kalbfleisch and Prentice (2002) described competing risks as the situation in which an individual can experience more than one type of event. Gelman *et al.* (1990) and Caplan *et al.* (1994) explain it as the failure to achieve independence between the time to an event and the censoring mechanism. And finally, Gooley *et al.* (1999) defined the concept of competing risks as the situation where one type of event 'either precludes the occurrence of another event under investigation or fundamentally alters the probability of occurrence of this other event'. This closely reflects the situation with which the clinical researcher or the applied statistician is faced: the possibility of many types of failure that compete with each other to be observed.

Suppose that a study of a new treatment for heart disease is carried out in an older population. Given the advanced age of the

Competing Risks: A Practical Perspective   M. Pintilie
© 2006 John Wiley & Sons, Ltd

study group it is possible, and perhaps likely, that a patient may die of a cause other than heart failure. A death due to some other cause constitutes a competing risk type of event, because it hinders the observation of the event of interest – death due to heart disease.

3.1.2   Common endpoints in medical research

This section begins with an illustration of endpoints that are commonly encountered in cancer studies. More general explanations and examples from other fields of medical research are also introduced.

In cancer research, patients undergo one or more of the three main types of treatment: surgery, chemotherapy and radiation therapy. Suppose that the treatment appeared successful and all evidence of disease was removed. A common endpoint of interest in cancer studies is the time to the return of disease (relapse) after the initial apparent success of treatment. The relapse may be at the site of the initial disease, in which case the endpoint is called *local relapse*, or at a different site, called *distant relapse* or metastasis.

Chemotherapy, as a systemic treatment, affects the whole body while both surgery and radiation therapies are treatments directed towards the specific disease site. Therefore, in studies of radiation or surgery, the researcher may be more interested in the time to local relapse than in the time to metastasis or death. In this case, it is desirable to identify characteristics that are associated with local relapse. However, a patient may develop distant disease and die before a local relapse is observed. In this case the observation of distant disease hinders the observation of local disease. Furthermore, the occurrence of local disease after distant disease may not be of much interest since treatment of the distant disease may alter the chances of local disease recurring.

More generally, the term 'relapse' refers to the return or recurrence of any potentially chronic condition or disease after an initial improvement. For instance, in studies of smoking cessation, relapse refers to the resumption of the previous smoking behaviour. Psychiatric studies of patients with bipolar disorder might consider a repeat episode of mania to be a relapse, while a clinical trial involving patients with chronic bronchitis might define a relapse to be the reappearance of the symptoms. Pulmonary tuberculosis could recur either within the lung (local relapse) or at extrapulmonary sites (other relapse). Similarly, a relapse of the herpes simplex virus could be experienced as a skin lesion (local relapse) or within the central nervous system (other relapse). Therefore, the concept of relapse (local, distant or other) is a meaningful endpoint in other medical areas, beside cancer, where the disease or condition under study may reappear at different sites within the body.

Without being exhaustive, Table 3.1 gives several endpoints and their definitions as they are used in this book. It also identifies possible competing risks associated with each of these endpoints.

3.2   TWO MATHEMATICAL DEFINITIONS

There are two mathematical approaches to dealing with competing risks, and both have received attention in the literature. In this section the two mathematical definitions of competing risks are introduced, as well as the main concepts: subdistribution, subdensity, subhazard, cause-specific hazard and the hazard of the subdistribution.

3.2.1   Competing risks as bivariate random variable

In the absence of competing risks, survival data are usually presented as a bivariate random variable or pair (T, C). The censoring variable, C, is 1 if the event of interest was observed, and is 0 if the observation was censored. When $C = 1$ the first member of the pair, T, is the time at which the event occurred and when $C = 0$, T is the time at which the observation was censored.

This definition can be extended to the competing risks situation where $p \geq 2$ types of failures or events are possible. The data are again represented as a pair (T, C), and the censoring indicator C will again be defined as 0 if the observation is censored. In the event that the observation is not censored, though, C will take on the value i, where i is the type of the first failure/event observed $(i = 1, 2, \ldots, p)$. If $C = i$ then T is the time at which the event of

Table 3.1 Examples of endpoints.

Endpoint	Measurement	Event of interest	Possible competing risks
Survival	Time to death from any cause	Death from any cause	No competing risks
Disease-free survival	Time to first failure: relapse or death	Relapse or death	No competing risks
Local relapse incidence	Time to local relapse	Local relapse	Relapse at other locations or death without local relapse
Distant relapse incidence	Time to distant relapse	Distant relapse	Relapse at other locations or death without distant relapse
Cause-specific survival	Time to death due to disease under study	Death due to disease under study	Death due to other causes
Incidence of non-fatal MI	Time to non-fatal MI	Non-fatal MI	Cardiovascular death and non-vascular death, non-fatal stroke and angina
Incidence of involuntary pregnancy	Time to involuntary pregnancy	Involuntary pregnancy	Other types of discontinuation of IUD (medical or non-medical removal, expulsion, other)

type i occurred; otherwise it is the time of censoring (Kalbfleisch and Prentice, 1980; Crowder, 2001).

In the hypoxia trial, T is the time to the first failure or censoring, whichever comes first, where the types of failure can be local relapse ($i = 1$), distant relapse ($i = 2$) or local and distant relapse together ($i = 3$).

Scrutinio *et al.* (2001) reported the results of a randomized, double-blinded multicentre trial on patients with myocardial infarction (MI) treated with either ticlopidine or aspirin. In this trial, T is defined as the time from randomization to the first failure. The types of failure and therefore the choices for C are cardiovascular death ($i = 1$), non-vascular death ($i = 2$), non-fatal MI ($i = 3$), non-fatal stroke ($i = 4$) and angina ($i = 5$).

3.2.2   Competing risks as latent failure times

The second mathematical definition of the competing risks outcome is written in terms of p latent, or unobserved, event times $T_1, T_2, \ldots, T_p$, one for each of the p event types. In the competing risks situation only the first event is observed, and so the time variable, T, is defined as the earliest of these hypothetical, unobserved times. Mathematically, then, $T = \min\{T_1, T_2, \ldots, T_p\}$. The censoring variable, C, is defined as $C = 0$ if the observation is censored, and $C = i$, $i = 1, 2, \ldots, p$, otherwise.

In the tamoxifen trial T_1 might be time to local relapse, T_2 time to distant relapse, T_3 time to other malignancy and T_4 time to death without any of these events. The observed time is $T = \min\{T_1, T_2, T_3, T_4\}$, and C is 1 when the first event is local relapse, 2 if the first event is distant relapse, 3 if malignancy was observed, 4 for death without events, and zero otherwise.

As a further illustration of the latent variables approach, consider the 1997 report by the World Health Organization on trials of intrauterine devices (IUDs) for contraception (Rowe *et al.*, 1997; Tai, 2001). The time variable was defined as time between randomization and the discontinuation of the device. The reasons for discontinuation were classified as: involuntary pregnancy, expulsion, medical reason for removal (due to pain, bleeding, infection), non-medical reason for removal (no further need or the wish to become pregnant) and other reasons. Since only one of the reasons could be observed the time variable is $T = \min\{T_1, T_2, T_3, T_4, T_5\}$, where T_1 is time to involuntary pregnancy, T_2 is time to expulsion, T_3 is time to medical removal, T_4 is time to non-medical removal, T_5 is time to other reasons for discontinuation, and $C = 1, 2, 3, 4$ or 5 depending on the event observed or $C = 0$ for censored observations.

3.3   FUNDAMENTAL CONCEPTS

There are several mathematical functions of importance in the competing risks setting: the subdistribution, subdensity, subhazard, cause-specific hazard and the hazard of the subdistribution. There has unfortunately been little agreement in terms of nomenclature, and readers consulting the literature will find these functions referred to by a number of other terms. For instance, the subdistribution has been referred to as the cumulative incidence function (Kalbfleisch and Prentice, 1980), the marginal distribution (Pepe and Mori, 1993), the absolute cause-specific risk (Benichou and Gail, 1990), the crude incidence curve (Korn and Dorey, 1992), and the cause-specific failure probability (Gaynor *et al.*, 1993). In this book the terms cumulative incidence function (CIF) and subdistribution are preferred. The former has been more consistently used throughout the literature, and the latter can often be found in theoretical contexts. This section is concerned with the definitions of these functions and the relationships between them.

3.3.1   Competing risks as bivariate random variable

The CIF, or subdistribution, for an event of type i $(i = 1, 2, \ldots, p)$ is defined as the joint probability

$$F_i(t) = P(T \leq t, C = i). \tag{3.1}$$

In other words, the CIF is the probability that an event of type i occurs at or before time t.

The overall distribution function is the probability that an event of any type occurs at or before time t. As exemplified in Figure 1.1, the overall distribution function is equal to the sum of CIFs, for all event types. Hence,

$$F(t) = P(T \le t) = \sum_{i=1}^{p} P(T \le t, C = i) = \sum_{i=1}^{p} F_i(t).$$

The subsurvivor function is the probability that an event of type i does not occur by time t and is defined as $S_i(t) = P(T > t, C = i)$. Note here that when the competing risks are not present the overall distribution function spans the interval $[0,1]$. In contrast, in the competing risks environment the CIF can take values only up to $P(C = i)$ because

$$\lim_{t \to \infty} F_i(t) = P(C = i).$$

Therefore, $F_i(t)$ is not a proper distribution, hence the term 'subdistribution'. Also note that

$$F_i(t) + S_i(t) = P(C = i).$$

In addition to the CIF and the subsurvivor function, the subdensity function for events of type i is defined as

$$f_i(t) = \frac{\partial F_i(t)}{\partial t}.$$

As in the general setting of survival analysis (Chapter 2), the subhazard can be defined in mathematical terms as

$$\tilde{h}_i(t) = \lim_{\delta t \to 0} \left\{ \frac{P(t < T \le t + \delta t, C = i | T > t)}{\delta t} \right\}. \qquad (3.2)$$

The subhazard has the same interpretation as the hazard in the non-competing risks setting – the instantaneous event rate. The overall hazard of an event of any type can be found by summing over all subhazards:

$$h(t) = \sum_{i=1}^{p} \tilde{h}_i(t)$$

It is worth pointing out that because the CIF is a joint probability, some of the relationships among the various subfunctions may not be as expected. Based on (2.3) one would expect that $\widetilde{h}_i(t) = f_i(t)/S_i(t)$. However, simplifying (3.2) gives

$$
\begin{aligned}
\widetilde{h}_i(t) &= \lim_{\delta t \to 0} \left\{ \frac{P(t < T \le t + \delta t, C = i | T > t)}{\delta t} \right\} \\
&= \lim_{\delta t \to 0} \left\{ \frac{P(t < T \le t + \delta t, C = i)}{\delta t P(T > t)} \right\} \\
&= \{P(T > t)\}^{-1} \lim_{\delta t \to 0} \left\{ \frac{P(t < T \le t + \delta t, C = i)}{\delta t} \right\} \\
&= \frac{f_i(t)}{S(t)}.
\end{aligned}
\tag{3.3}
$$

In contrast, the hazard function of the subdistribution (Gray, 1988) is defined as

$$
\gamma_i(t) = \lim_{\delta t \to 0} \left\{ \frac{P(t < T \le t + \delta t, C = i | T > t \text{ or } (T \le t \text{ and } C \ne i))}{\delta t} \right\}.
$$

The relationship between $\gamma_i(t)$ and the subdensity and the subdistribution can be expressed as

$$
\gamma_i(t) = \frac{f_i(t)}{1 - F_i(t)}.
\tag{3.4}
$$

The cumulative subhazard function is defined as

$$
H_i(t) = \int_0^t h_i(x)dx = \int_0^t \{f_i(x)/S(x)\} \, dx.
$$

The material presented in this book is concerned primarily with nonparametric or semiparametric methods, which are more fully developed in the literature. However, parametric distributions are also used for modelling competing risks data, and several are considered here. Table 3.2 gives the functions defined in this section for several parametric distributions, when only two types of events are possible: type 1 is the event of interest and type 2 is the competing risk. This does not restrict the generality because all types of events other than the event of interest can be grouped together as a single competing risk.

Table 3.2 Parametric models: bivariate approach.

Distribution	Subsurvivor function	Cumulative incidence function	Subdensity function	Subhazard function	Hazard function of subdistribution
Mixture of exponentials	$p_1 e^{-\lambda_1 t}$	$p_1\left(1 - e^{-\lambda_1 t}\right)$	$p_1 \lambda_1 e^{-\lambda_1 t}$	$\dfrac{p_1 \lambda_1 e^{-\lambda_1 t}}{p_1 e^{-\lambda_1 t} + p_2 e^{-\lambda_2 t}}$	$\dfrac{p_1 \lambda_1 e^{-\lambda_1 t}}{1 - p_1\left(1 - e^{-\lambda_1 t}\right)}$
Mixture of Weibulls*	$p_1 e^{-\Lambda_1(t,\alpha_1)}$	$p_1\left(1 - e^{-\Lambda_1(t,\alpha_1)}\right)$	$p_1 \lambda_1 \alpha_1 \Lambda\left(t,\alpha_1 - 1\right) e^{-\Lambda_1(t,\alpha_1)}$	$\dfrac{p_1 \lambda_1 \alpha_1 \Lambda\left(t,\alpha_1 - 1\right) e^{-\Lambda_1(t,\alpha_1)}}{p_1 e^{-\Lambda_1(t,\alpha_1)} + p_2 e^{-\Lambda_2(t,\alpha_2)}}$	$\dfrac{p_1 \lambda_1 \alpha_1 \Lambda\left(t,\alpha_1 - 1\right) e^{-\Lambda_1(t,\alpha_1)}}{1 - p_1\left(1 - e^{-\Lambda_1(t,\alpha_1)}\right)}$
Independent Weibulls	No closed form	No closed form	$\alpha_1 \lambda_1^{\alpha_1} t^{\alpha_1 - 1} e^{-\left\{(\lambda_1 t)^{\alpha_1} + (\lambda_2 t)^{\alpha_2}\right\}}$	$\alpha_1 \lambda_1^{\alpha_1} t^{\alpha_1 - 1}$	No closed form

*$\Lambda_1\left(t,\alpha_1\right) = \left(\lambda_1 t\right)^{\alpha_1}$.

The first row in Table 3.2 corresponds to a mixture of exponential distributions, while the second row is a natural extension of the exponential mixture to a Weibull mixture. The third row corresponds to a second Weibull-based distribution. In this case, the subhazard is defined first and the CIF does not have a closed form (Crowder, 2001). The distributions included in Table 3.2 were chosen because they have relatively simple mathematical forms and have appeared in the literature as providing reasonable models for many cases of competing risks data.

3.3.2   Competing risks as latent failure times

Since the latent variables approach is based on a collection of p latent times, let us begin by defining the multivariate joint survivor function

$$S\left(t_1, t_2, \ldots, t_p\right) = P\left(T_1 > t_1, T_2 > t_2, \ldots, T_p > t_p\right).$$

Then the subdensity for event type i is

$$f_i(t) = \left(-\frac{\partial S\left(t_1, t_2, \ldots, t_p\right)}{\partial t_i}\right)_{t_1 = t_2 = \ldots = t_p = t}.$$

The marginal survivor function for event type i is

$$S_i(t) = S\left(t_1 = 0, t_2 = 0, \ldots, t_i = t, \ldots, t_p = 0\right),$$

and the subdistribution function is defined as follows:

$$F_j(t) = \int_0^t f_j(s) ds. \tag{3.5}$$

The subdistribution function represents the probability of an event of type i happening by time t.

The approach to deriving the subhazard is the same as for the bivariate approach, and after some algebra it can be shown that

$$\widetilde{h}_i(t) = \left(-\frac{\partial \log\left(S\left(t_1, t_2, \ldots, t_p\right)\right)}{\partial t_i}\right)_{t_1 = t_2 = \ldots = t_p = t} \tag{3.6}$$

The cause-specific hazard is defined as the hazard of the marginal distribution,

$$h_i(t) = -\frac{\partial \log (S_i(t))}{\partial t} = \frac{f_i(t)}{S_i(t)}, \tag{3.7}$$

and in the case where the p latent times are statistically independent, it is identical to the subhazard. For the examples given in the Table 3.3 the cause-specific hazard is the same as the subhazard except for the second example where the cause-specific hazard is still λ_1 as for the independent case. Note that the cause specific hazard is defined only in the latent failure time approach of competing risks.

The definition of the hazard of the subdistribution is the same as in the bivariate distribution framework.

Table 3.3 gives the joint and marginal survivor functions, CIF, subdensity and subhazard functions for several parametric distributions. As before, the examples are presented assuming that only two types of event are possible: the event of interest (type 1) and the competing risk (type 2).

3.3.3 Discussion of the two approaches

To many, the definition based on latent failure times seems more intuitive than the bivariate approach, and it is appealing for that reason. However, one major disadvantage of the latent failure times approach is the issue of non-identifiability. This means that for the same two marginal distributions there is more than one joint distribution that can be defined. In other words, the marginal distributions do not define the joint distribution. However, when independence can be assumed between the distributions of the two event types the two marginals do uniquely define the joint distribution. The assumption of independence is a strong one, though, and can rarely be justified in real life. Unfortunately, when only the first event is observed this assumption cannot be tested. This means that the analysis based on latent failure times cannot make use of the possible dependence between the

Table 3.3 Parametric models: latent failure times approach.

Distribution	Joint survivor function	Marginal survivor function	Cumulative incidence function	Subdensity function	Subhazard function	Cause-specific hazard
Exponential independent	$e^{-(\lambda_1 t_1 + \lambda_2 t_2)}$	$e^{-\lambda_1 t}$	$\frac{\lambda_1}{\lambda_1+\lambda_2} \times (1 - e^{-(\lambda_1+\lambda_2)t})$	$\lambda_1 e^{-(\lambda_1+\lambda_2)t}$	λ_1	λ_1
Exponential dependent	$e^{-(\lambda_1 t_1 + \lambda_2 t_2 + \nu t_1 t_2)}$	$e^{-\lambda_1 t}$	$\frac{1}{2}\left\{1 - e^{-(\lambda_1 t + \lambda_2 t + \nu t^2)} + G(\lambda_1,\lambda_2,\nu,t)\right\}^{*}$	$(\lambda_1 + \nu t)\, e^{-(\lambda_1 t + \lambda_2 t + \nu t^2)}$	$\lambda_1 + \nu t$	λ_1
Weibull independent	$e^{-\{(\lambda_1 t_1)^{\alpha_1} + (\lambda_2 t_2)^{\alpha_2}\}}$	$e^{-(\lambda_1 t)^{\alpha_1}}$	$\frac{\lambda_1^{\alpha}}{\lambda_1^{\alpha}+\lambda_2^{\alpha}} \times (1 - e^{-(\lambda_1^{\alpha}+\lambda_2^{\alpha})t^{\alpha}})^{\ddagger}$	$\lambda_1 \alpha_1 (\lambda_1 t)^{\alpha_1 - 1}\, e^{-\{(\lambda_1 t)^{\alpha_1} + (\lambda_2 t)^{\alpha_2}\}}$	$\lambda_1 \alpha_1 (\lambda_1 t)^{\alpha_1 - 1}$	$\lambda_1 \alpha_1 (\lambda_1 t)^{\alpha_1 - 1}$
Marshall–Olkin	$e^{-(\lambda_1 t_1 + \lambda_2 t_2 + \mu \max(t_1,t_2))}$	$e^{-(\lambda_1 + \mu)t}$	$\frac{\lambda_1+\mu}{\lambda_1+\lambda_2+\mu} \times (1 - e^{-(\lambda_1+\lambda_2+\mu)t})$	$(\lambda_1 + \mu)\, e^{-(\lambda_1+\lambda_2+\mu)t}$	$\lambda_1 + \mu$	$\lambda_1 + \mu$

$^{*}G(\lambda_1, \lambda_2, \nu, t) = (\lambda_1 - \lambda_2)\sqrt{\frac{\pi}{\nu}}\exp\left\{\frac{(\lambda_1+\lambda_2)^2}{4\nu}\right\}\left\{\frac{1}{2} - \Phi\left(-\sqrt{2\nu}\left[t + \frac{\lambda_1+\lambda_2}{2\nu}\right]\right)\right\}$, where Φ is the standard normal distribution function.

$^{\ddagger}\alpha_1 = \alpha_2 = \alpha.$

times to different types of event. The undesirable effect of non-identifiability is apparent in Table 3.3. The marginal survivor functions of the first two examples are the same, although the joint survivor functions are different. The second row represents a joint distribution corresponding to two dependent exponential distributions. The parameter ν expresses the level of dependency. In contrast, in the first example $\nu = 0$ and the two distributions are independent. In fact, there are multitudes of joint distributions that produce the same marginals (Tsiatis, 1975). For this case the definition of competing risks based on the latent failure time loses some of its appeal: one cannot model, estimate, or test for the dependence between the times to different types of failures.

When the latent failure time definition is considered one can only model the marginal distribution function and the cause-specific hazard (3.7). Cox and Oakes (1984) note that the cause-specific hazard can always be estimated without the special assumption of independence. This assumption is essential for the estimation of the joint survivor function.

From this point on, the term 'cause-specific hazard' refers to the hazard of the marginal distribution in the sense of latent failure time definition. Only the cause-specific hazard and the hazard of the subdistribution are used in modelling and testing. The term 'subhazard' will mean only the subhazard in the sense of the bivariate definition.

Note that the subhazard depends on the parameters of the competing risks but the cause-specific hazard does not.

3.4 CLOSING REMARKS

This chapter has introduced the idea of competing risks in medical research. The latter part of the chapter is concerned with the mathematical definitions of competing risks and the main theoretical concepts are defined. Readers interested in greater theoretical detail are referred to Crowder (2001).

The nonparametric estimation of the CIF is presented in the next chapter, while the comparison of CIFs is discussed in Chapter 5. When the competing risks are ignored and the usual survival techniques are used, the marginal distribution and therefore its hazard (the cause-specific hazard, (3.7)) are modelled. An extension of the Cox proportional hazards model to account for competing risks was introduced by Fine and Gray (1999) where the parameter which is modelled is the hazard of the subdistribution (3.4).

4

Descriptive methods for competing risks data

4.1 PRODUCT-LIMIT ESTIMATOR AND COMPETING RISKS

For survival analysis when there is a single event of interest and no competing risks, the product-limit estimator (Kaplan–Meier estimator) is frequently used in describing the time-to-event experience of the subjects under study. It is straightforward to calculate, lends itself well to graphical depiction, and can be easily understood by clinical and other researchers. It seems natural to apply the same technique when competing risks are present. Indeed, many research papers have appeared in which the Kaplan–Meier estimate has been applied in this situation. However, its interpretation in the presence of competing risks is different.

Consider a hypothetical example of a study of 20 patients for which the time to discharge from hospital was recorded. The event of interest is time to discharge and the competing risk is death prior to discharge. All 20 patients were observed until the time of their discharge, or until they died, so there were no censored observations. The data are presented in Table 4.1. The joint probability that an event occurs within one month (30 days) and

Competing Risks: A Practical Perspective   M. Pintilie
© 2006 John Wiley & Sons, Ltd

Table 4.1 Discharge or death data.

Patient ID	Time to hospital discharge or death (days)	Type of event*
1	1	2
2	2	2
3	3	2
4	4	1
5	5	2
6	7	2
7	8	1
8	10	2
9	13	1
10	14	2
11	15	1
12	17	2
13	20	1
14	30	1
15	42	1
16	50	1
17	65	1
18	80	2
19	84	1
20	90	1

*1 = Discharge from hospital, 2 = Death.

that the event is discharge from hospital can be easily calculated. An empirical estimate of the probability of discharge from hospital by 30 days, $F_1(30) = P(T \leq 30, C = 1)$, is

$$\hat{F}_1(30) = \frac{\text{Number of patients discharged by 30 days}}{\text{Total number of patients}} = \frac{6}{20} = 0.30.$$

In this formula, T denotes the time to the patient's first event, discharge from hospital or death, and C stands for the type of event, with $C = 1$ for discharge from hospital and $C = 2$ for death.

The Kaplan–Meier estimate, on the other hand, depends on the order in which the discharges and deaths occurred relative to each other. For this example, the Kaplan–Meier estimate at 30 days obtained by treating the deaths as censored is

$$\hat{S}(30) = 1 \times \frac{16}{17} \times \frac{13}{14} \times \frac{11}{12} \times \frac{9}{10} \times \frac{7}{8} \times \frac{6}{7} = 0.54.$$

Using this estimate to calculate the probability of discharge from hospital by 30 days gives $\tilde{F}_1(30) = 1 - 0.54 = 0.46$, a considerably larger estimate than $\hat{F}_1(30) = 0.30$. $\tilde{F}_1(t)$ estimates the probability of discharge from hospital by 30 days but ignoring the possibility that some individuals die before discharge.

Given that the Kaplan–Meier estimate ignores events of all types other than the one of interest, it can be interpreted as the probability of an event beyond time t given that all other risks were removed. However, in many medical settings this may be a nonsensical interpretation. If, for example, the event of interest was relapse of breast cancer in the presence of the competing risk of death due to non-relapse-related causes, then one would be forced to consider the unrealistic case where death due to all non-relapse-related causes was eliminated.

In fact the Kaplan–Meier method estimates the function $\exp\left\{-\int_0^t h_1(u)du\right\}$, where $h_1(u)$ is the cause-specific hazard function obtained by treating the competing risks as censored.

To estimate the probability of an event Kalbfleisch and Prentice (1980, 2002) suggest using the cumulative incidence function, which is presented in Section 4.2. Section 4.3 illustrates by example how to obtain these estimates using SAS and R.

4.2 CUMULATIVE INCIDENCE FUNCTION

In this section we derive the nonparametric estimation of the cumulative incidence function (CIF) and two estimates of its variance. We first present a heuristic derivation of the CIF in Section 4.2.1, followed by a more rigorous approach in Section 4.2.2. There is a moderate amount of mathematics involved in the latter, some of which is given here. Some readers may wish to skip Section 4.2.2 as it is not essential in understanding the concept of the CIF.

4.2.1   Heuristic estimation of the CIF

In the case where there is no censoring, an empirical estimate of the CIF for the event of type i can be obtained as

$$\hat{F}_i(t) = \frac{\text{Number of observations with } T \le t \text{ and } C = i}{n},$$

where n is the total number of observations.

However, if among the n observations some did not yet experience any of the p types of events, then censored observations are present in the dataset. Let $t_1 < t_2 < \ldots < t_r$ be the unique ordered uncensored time points. Define d_{ij} to be the number of events of type i that occur at time t_j. An individual is at risk at t_j if his observed time, censored or not, is t_j or larger. The number at risk at t_j is denoted by n_j. $\hat{S}(t)$ is the Kaplan–Meier estimator of the probability of being free of any event by time t. The CIF can be calculated as the sum over all t_j of the probabilities of observing event i at time t_j, while the individual is still at risk: that is to say, the individual did not experience any event prior to t_j. The probability of remaining event-free prior to t_j is $\hat{S}(t_{j-1})$. It follows that the joint probability of being event-free immediately prior to t_j and experiencing an event of type i at t_j is

$$\hat{F}_i(t) = \sum_{\text{all } j, t_j \le t} \hat{h}_{ij} \hat{S}(t_{j-1}), \qquad (4.1)$$

where h_{ij} is the cause-specific hazard for event i at t_j. Intuitively, given that an individual has not experienced an event of any type up to t_{j-1}, the probability of an event of type i in the interval $t_j - \delta$ to t_j can be estimated as d_{ij}/n_j. It follows that

$$\hat{F}_i(t) = \sum_{\text{all } j, t_j \le t} \frac{d_{ij}}{n_j} \hat{S}(t_{j-1}). \qquad (4.2)$$

Thus, the CIF estimator for an event of type i depends not only on the number of individuals who have experienced this type of event, but also on the number of individuals who have not experienced any other type of event. The CIF represents the probability that an individual will experience an event of type i by time t.

It can be proven that at any time point, t_k, the complement of the Kaplan–Meier estimate $(1 - KM)$ is larger than the estimate of the CIF. Without any loss of generality, suppose that there are two types of event: the event of interest, denoted by subscript 1, and the set of competing risk events, denoted by subscript 2. Algebraically, the Kaplan–Meier estimate can be written as

$$KM_1(t_k) = \prod_{j=1}^{k} \frac{n_j - d_{1j}}{n_j}$$

$$= \frac{n_k - d_{1k}}{n_k} KM_1(t_{k-1})$$

$$= KM_1(t_{k-1}) - \frac{d_{1k}}{n_k} KM_1(t_{k-1}).$$

This implies that

$$1 - KM_1(t_k) = 1 - KM_1(t_{k-1}) + \frac{d_{1k}}{n_k} KM_1(t_{k-1})$$

$$= \sum_{j=1}^{k} \frac{d_{1j}}{n_j} KM_1(t_{j-1}).$$

This formula can be compared with the formula for the estimate of the CIF written for the event of interest:

$$\hat{F}_1(t) = \sum_{j-1}^{k} \frac{d_{1j}}{n_j} \hat{S}(t_{j-1}).$$

The value KM_1 is the Kaplan–Meier estimate when only the event of interest is used, while $\hat{S}$ is the Kaplan–Meier estimate when all events (the event of interest as well as competing risk events) are considered. Thus, $\hat{S}(t) \leq KM_1(t)$ for any t. The equality happens when there are no competing risk events. It follows that $\hat{F}_1(t_k) \leq 1 - KM_1(t_k)$.

In the context of studies involving cancer treatment where the competing events are local relapse, distant relapse, and death without disease, the overall Kaplan–Meier estimate $\hat{S}(t)$ is often called *disease-free survival*.

4.2.2   Nonparametric maximum likelihood estimation of the CIF

In this section a rigorous estimator for h_{ij}, and therefore for the subdistribution function, is derived. The notation of Section 4.2.1 is retained, and it is also assumed that in the interval $[t_{j-1}, t_j)$ there are m_j censored observations at time points $t_{j1} < t_{j2} < \ldots < t_{jm_j}$. The likelihood function can be written as

$$L = \left[\prod_{j=1}^{r} \prod_{i=1}^{p} \{F_i(t_j) - F_i(t_{j-1})\}^{d_{ij}} \right] \left[\prod_{j=1}^{r+1} \prod_{l=1}^{m_j} S(t_{jl}) \right]$$

or, in terms of the cause-specific hazard,

$$L = \prod_{j=1}^{r} \prod_{i=1}^{p} h_{ij}^{d_{ij}} (1 - h_j)^{n_j - d_j},$$

where h_j is the hazard of any type of event at time t_j.

As usual, the log-likelihood is differentiated with respect to h_{ij} and the derivative is set to zero. The following equation is obtained:

$$h_{ij} = \frac{d_{ij}(1 - h_j)}{n_j - d_j}. \tag{4.3}$$

Since $h_j = \sum_{i=1}^{p} h_{ij}$ and $d_j = \sum_{i=1}^{p} d_{ij}$, equation (4.3) becomes

$$h_j = \frac{d_j(1 - h_j)}{n_j - d_j}$$

and the estimator for h_j is $\hat{h}_j = d_j/n_j$. Replacing this formula in (4.3), one obtains $\hat{h}_{ij} = d_{ij}/n_j$ which, substituted in (4.1), gives the CIF estimator as

$$\hat{F}_i(t) = \sum_{t_j \leq t} \frac{d_{ij}}{n_j} \hat{S}(t_{j-1}),$$

where $\hat{S}(t)$ is the Kaplan–Meier estimator that would have been obtained by considering all events to be of the same type. As expected, the maximum likelihood estimate of the CIF is the same as that obtained through heuristic arguments presented earlier in Section 4.2.1.

4.2.3   Calculating the CIF estimator

The following hypothetical example is introduced to illustrate the calculation of the CIF estimator. Suppose that a study of falling in elderly patients at a particular rehabilitation institution included 10 subjects. The event of interest was an injurious fall that resulted in delayed rehabilitation. In this example, there are two competing risks: death and discharge from the institution. Only the number of days to the first event was recorded. The data are given in Table 4.2. The censoring variable is coded as 0 if no event was observed, 1 for an injurious fall, 2 for death, and 3 for discharge from hospital.

Table 4.3 illustrates the calculations using equation (4.2). $\hat{S}(t)$ is the estimate of the survivor function when all types of events are considered and is calculated using the Kaplan–Meier method. $\hat{F}_1(t)$, $\hat{F}_2(t)$ and $\hat{F}_3(t)$ are the respective estimates for the probability of an event of each type (CIF): injurious fall, death and discharge from hospital. The hazard estimate for each event type is calculated at each of the event times, and, together with $\hat{S}(t)$, it is used to obtain the estimate of the corresponding CIF.

From the calculations in Table 4.3, the estimated probability that an individual will experience an injurious fall before 3 months (90 days) is $\hat{F}_1(90) = \hat{F}_1(80) = 0.2250$. Similarly, the probability of death by 3 months is $\hat{F}_2(90) = 0.2125$, and the probability of discharge from hospital is $\hat{F}_3(90) = 0.2250$. The curves are plotted in Figure 4.1.

The probability of observing an event of any type was partitioned into three probabilities, one for each type of event (Figure 4.2):

$$\hat{F}_1(t) + \hat{F}_2(t) + \hat{F}_3(t) = 1 - \hat{S}(t).$$

Table 4.2   Injurious fall data.

Subject ID	101	102	103	104	105	106	107	108	109	110
Time to the first event (days)	128	80	61	24	113	65	106	37	80	49
Type of event*	1	1	2	2	0	3	2	0	3	1

* 0 = Censored, 1 = Injurious fall, 2 = Death, 3 = Discharge from hospital.

Table 4.3 Calculating the CIF

Time to event	Type of event	n at risk	$\hat{S}(t)$	$\hat{F}_1(t)$	$\hat{F}_2(t)$	$\hat{F}_3(t)$
0	–	10	1.0000	0.0000	0.0000	0.0000
24	2	10	$1-1/10 = 0.9000$	$1 \times 0/10 = 0.0000$	0.1000	0.0000
37	0	9	0.9000	$0 + 0.9 \times 0/9 = 0.0000$	0.1000	0.0000
49	1	8	$0.9000(1-1/8) = 0.7875$	$0 + 0.9 \times 1/8 = 0.1125$	0.1000	0.0000
61	2	7	$0.7875(1-1/7) = 0.6750$	$0.1125 + 0.7875 \times 0/7 = 0.1125$	0.2125	0.0000
65	3	6	$0.6750(1-1/6) = 0.5625$	$0.1125 + 0.675 \times 0/6 = 0.1125$	0.2125	0.1125
80	1	5	$0.5625(1-2/5) = 0.3375$	$0.1125 + 0.5625 \times 1/5 = 0.2250$	0.2125	0.2250
80	3					
106	2	3	$0.3375(1-1/3) = 0.2250$	$0.2250 + 0.3375 \times 0/3 = 0.2250$	0.3250	0.2250
113	0	2	0.2250	$0.2250 + 0.225 \times 0/2 = 0.2250$	0.3250	0.2250
128	1	1	$0.2250(1-1/1) = 0.0000$	$0.2250 + 0.225 \times 1/1 = 0.4500$	0.3250	0.2250

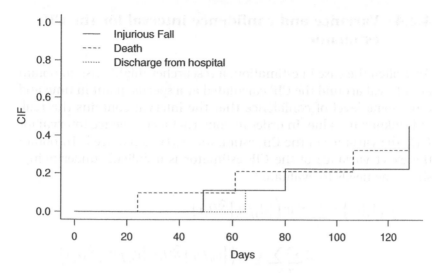

Figure 4.1 Estimated CIF for the three types of events.

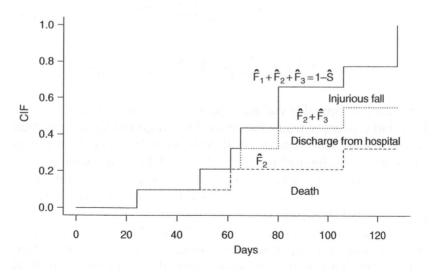

Figure 4.2 Partition of the $1 - \hat{S}(t)$ into $\hat{F}_1(t), \hat{F}_2(t)$ and $\hat{F}_3(t)$.

4.2.4   Variance and confidence interval for the CIF estimator

As is often the case in estimation, a researcher might wish to obtain an interval around the CIF calculated at a specific point in time and have some level of confidence that the interval contains the real, but unknown, value. In order to construct a confidence interval for $F_i(t)$ the variance of the CIF estimator, $\hat{F}_i(t)$, is required. To obtain the exact variance of the CIF estimator is a difficult undertaking, since one needs to evaluate

$$V\left(\hat{F}_i(t)\right) = \sum_{t_j \leq t} \text{Var}\left(\{d_{ij}/n_j\}\hat{S}(t_j)\right)$$

$$+ 2\sum_{t_j < t}\sum_{\substack{t_v > t_j \\ t_v \leq t}} \text{Cov}\left(\{d_{ij}/n_j\}\hat{S}(t_j), \{d_{iv}/n_v\}\hat{S}(t_v)\right).$$

Using the delta method, $V\left(\hat{F}_i(t)\right)$ can be estimated as:

$$\hat{V}_{\text{DM}}\left(\hat{F}_i(t)\right) = \sum_{t_j \leq t}\left\{\left[\hat{F}_i(t) - \hat{F}_i(t_j)\right]^2 \frac{d_j}{n_j\left(n_j - d_j\right)}\right\}$$

$$+ \sum_{t_j \leq t}\hat{S}(t_{j-1})^2\frac{d_{ij}\left(n_j - d_{ij}\right)}{n_j^3} \qquad (4.4)$$

$$- 2\sum_{t_j \leq t}\left[\hat{F}_i(t) - \hat{F}_i(t_j)\right]\hat{S}(t_{j-1})\frac{d_{ij}}{n_j^2}.$$

The details of how this variance estimator is obtained are not given here, but readers who are interested in its mathematical derivation can find it in Marubini and Valsecchi (1995). Since $\hat{F}_i$ is a step function, terms that include $\hat{F}_i(t) - \hat{F}_i(t_j)$ will be 0 unless an event of type i has occurred between times t_j and t. Likewise, terms involving d_{ij} will be 0 except at those time points where an event of type i has been recorded. Therefore the last term of each sum is non-zero only if at time t there is an event of type i. When there is only one type of event and no competing risks, formula (4.4) for the estimated variance is identical to Greenwood's formula for the usual survival analysis setting (formula (2.7)).

The variance estimator may also be derived using the work of Aalen (1978a) as follows:

$$
\hat{V}_A\left(\hat{F}_i(t)\right) = \sum_{t_j \le t} \left\{ \left[\hat{F}_i(t) - \hat{F}_i(t_j)\right]^2 \frac{d_j}{(n_j-1)(n_j-d_j)} \right\}
$$

$$
+ \sum_{t_j \le t} \hat{S}(t_{j-1})^2 \frac{d_{ij}(n_j-d_{ij})}{n_j^2(n_j-1)} \tag{4.5}
$$

$$
- 2 \sum_{t_j \le t} \left[\hat{F}_i(t) - \hat{F}_i(t_j)\right] \hat{S}(t_{j-1}) \frac{d_{ij}(n_j-d_{ij})}{n_j(n_j-d_j)(n_j-1)}.
$$

An approximate $100(1-\alpha)\%$ confidence interval for the CIF for the event of interest, $F(t)$, based on its asymptotic normality, is

$$
\hat{F}(t) \pm z_{1-\alpha/2} \sqrt{\hat{V}\left(\hat{F}(t)\right)}, \tag{4.6}
$$

where z_α is the α quantile of the standard normal distribution and $\hat{V}$ is the variance estimator of the CIF. While this confidence interval has the advantage of being familiar and simple to construct, it has the unfortunate property that it may result in the bounds being negative or above 1. As shown in Section 2.3, this side effect can be avoided by finding a confidence interval for $\log\left(-\log\left(\hat{F}(t)\right)\right)$ first and transforming the bounds back to their original scale. The resulting confidence interval is of the form

$$
\hat{F}(t)^{\exp[\pm A]}, \tag{4.7}
$$

where

$$
A = \frac{z_{1-\alpha/2} \sqrt{\hat{V}(\hat{F}(t))}}{\hat{F}(t) \log\left(\hat{F}(t)\right)}.
$$

4.3 SOFTWARE AND EXAMPLES

4.3.1 Using R

This section illustrates how to use R software to obtain estimates for the CIF, together with their variance, confidence intervals and to produce graphs for the CIFs. It is assumed that the R software and the `cmprsk` package are already installed (Sections B.1.1 and B.1.5). The datasets can be downloaded from the website address given in the Preface and saved on the local drive, for example in C:/datasets. The reader can also download the functions and macros included in Sections B.3 and B.4 from the same website address. The bone marrow transplant study, described in Section 1.6.4, is used. The time to each type of event was recorded. For this section only the time to the first observed events is considered. The three types of events are: chronic graft versus host disease (CGVHD), relapse and death. First, the data need to be imported from the downloaded comma delimited file `bmt.txt`. The names of the variables are on the first line. As shown in Appendix B, the file can be read using:

```
> bmt=read.table('c:/datasets/bmt.txt',sep=',',header=T)
> names(bmt)
 [1]  "dx"        "tx"        "extent"    "agvhdgd"   "age"
 [6]  "survtime"  "reltime"   "agvhtime"  "cgvhtime"  "stat"
[11]  "rcens"     "agvh"      "cgvh"      "stnum"
```

Columns 6,7 and 9 contain the time to death, relapse and CGVHD calculated in years (`survtime, reltime, cgvhtime`) and the respective indicator variables are in columns 10,11 and 13 (`stat, rcens, cgvh`). The earliest time that any of these events happened is calculated by taking the minimum of the observed times:

```
> bmt$dftime=apply(cbind(bmt$cgvhtime, bmt$reltime,
  bmt$survtime),1,min)
```

The censoring variable `cens` is coded as 0 when no events were observed, 1 if CGVHD was observed as first event, 2 if a relapse was observed as the first event and 3 if death occurred before either of the events:

```
> cens=(bmt$dftime==bmt$cgvhtime & bmt$cgvh==1)+
+ 2*(bmt$dftime==bmt$reltime & bmt$rcens==1)+
+ 3*(bmt$dftime==bmt$survtime & bmt$stat==1)
```

To summarize the number of patients in each category use the command:

```
> table(cens)
cens
0  1 2 3
4 86 5 5
```

There are 4 patients for whom no event was observed, 86 for whom the first event was CGVHD, 5 with relapse as first event and 5 who died before the occurrence of any other type of event. In this dataset there were no patients with more than 1 type of event observed at the same time point.

As mentioned in Appendix B, the cmprsk library must be loaded by typing:

```
> library(cmprsk)

Loading required package: survival
Loading required package: splines
```

The function cuminc calculates the CIF estimates for type of event together with the variance based on Aalen's work given in formula (4.5):

```
> fit=cuminc(bmt$dftime,cens)
> fit
Estimates and Variances:
$est
                  0.5            1           1.5            2           2.5
1   1     0.68686869   0.85858586   0.85858586   0.87878788   0.87878788
1   2     0.05050505   0.05050505   0.05050505   0.05050505   0.05050505
1   3     0.05050505   0.05050505   0.05050505   0.05050505   0.05050505

$var
                  0.5            1           1.5            2           2.5
1 1   0.0022255131   0.0012926194   0.0012926194   0.0014077527   0.0014077527
1 2   0.0004926906   0.0004926906   0.0004926906   0.0004926906   0.0004926906
1 3   0.0004895710   0.0004895710   0.0004895710   0.0004895710   0.0004895710
```

The output under $est gives the estimates for CIF. The first column identifies the group. In this example the estimates for the whole group are calculated, and since there is just one stratum, it is automatically marked as 1. The second column represents the type of event according to the codes used in the cens variable. CGVHD was coded as 1, relapse as 2 and death as 3. Hence, the first line gives the probability for CGVHD at 0.5, 1, 1.5, 2, 2.5 years. The second line provides the estimates for the probability of relapse and the third line gives the estimates for the probability of death without relapse or GVHD. Thus the CIF of GVHD at 1 years is 0.86 and the CIFs of relapse and death at 1 year are both 0.05. In the same way $var contains the variance estimates for the three types of events at each time point.

The CIF estimates at 3, 6, 9 and 12 months (0.25, 0.5, 0.75 and 1 year) can be obtained using timepoints:

```
> timepoints(fit,times=c(0.25,0.5,0.75,1))
$est
                0.25          0.5         0.75            1
1   1   0.00000000   0.68686869   0.78787879   0.85858586
1   2   0.01010101   0.05050505   0.05050505   0.05050505
1   3   0.04040404   0.05050505   0.05050505   0.05050505

$var
                 0.25            0.5           0.75              1
1   1   0.0000000000   0.0022255131   0.0017480615   0.0012926194
1   2   0.0001020519   0.0004926906   0.0004926906   0.0004926906
1   3   0.0003957140   0.0004895710   0.0004895710   0.0004895710
```

The function cifDM given in Appendix B calculates the variance based on the delta method for the CIF for the event of interest. Hence, the cens variable needs to be modified to contain only the code for the event of interest (say 1 for CGVHD) and the code for the competing risk (2 for both relapse and death). First these changes must be made:

```
> cens2=cens
> cens2[cens2==3]=2
```

and the function

```
> fit2=cifDM(bmt$dftime,cens2)
```

can be applied. The results can be listed by typing fit2 at the prompt.

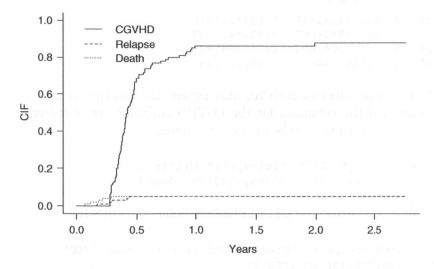

Figure 4.3 CIF estimates for the three types of events in the bone marrow transplant study.

To plot the CIF curves one can use the `plot.cuminc` function. The first parameter is a list which gives the time and the estimates produced with `cuminc`. The resulting plot is Figure 4.3.

```
> plot.cuminc(fit, ylab='CIF',
curvlab=c('CGHVD','Relapse','Death'))
```

To create a plot only for CGHVD for the two treatment arms: BM and PB, we first use `cuminc` to obtain the estimates:

```
> fit=cuminc(bmt$dftime,cens,bmt$tx)
> timepoints(fit,times=c(0.5,0.75))
$est
                0.5           0.75
BM   1    0.64000000    0.76000000
PB   1    0.73469388    0.81632653
BM   2    0.06000000    0.06000000
PB   2    0.04081633    0.04081633
BM   3    0.08000000    0.08000000
PB   3    0.02040816    0.02040816

$var
                0.5           0.75
BM   1   0.0048199634   0.0038954715
PB   1   0.0042011731   0.0033080316
```

```
BM   2   0.0011541610    0.0011541610
PB   2   0.0008436587    0.0008436587
BM   3   0.0015041822    0.0015041822
PB   3   0.0004164931    0.0004164931
```

Note that the label for each line also includes the label for treatment. Since only the estimates for the CGVHD endpoint are of interest, the proper list needs to be created by typing:

```
x=list(list(fit$'BM 1'$time,fit$'BM 1'$est),
       list(fit$'PB 1'$time,fit$'PB 1'$est))
```

and then applying the `plot.cuminc` function to this list:

```
plot.cuminc(x,xlab='Time to CGVHD (years)',ylab='CIF',
       curvlab=c('BM','PB'))
```

The graph is given in Figure 4.4.

Table 4.4 gives the 95% confidence intervals for the CIF for CGVHD at 0.5 years using Aalen estimates, the delta method and the two ways of deriving the confidence intervals (formulae

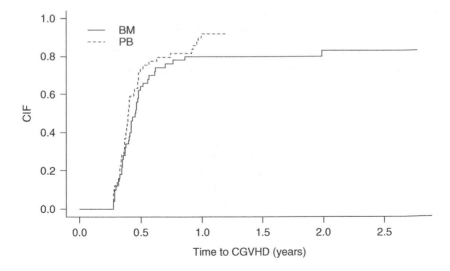

Figure 4.4 CIF for the CGVHD by treatment arms in the bone marrow transplant study.

Table 4.4 Ninety-five per cent confidence intervals for the CIF estimate for CGVHD at 0.5 years.

	CI based on (4.6)	CI based on (4.7)
Variance based on (4.4)	0.5955–0.7782	0.5855–0.7683
Variance based on (4.5)	0.5944–0.7793	0.5842–0.7691

(4.6) and (4.7). It is apparent from Table 4.4 that the differences are minimal. The confidence intervals based on (4.7) are not symmetrical in order to accommodate the situations when the estimate is very close to either 0 or 1.

4.3.2 Using SAS

The current version of SAS (Version 9) does not have any preprogrammed utilities for summarizing competing risks data. Appendix B includes two SAS macros that can be used for this purpose. The macro `cuminc` computes the estimates of the CIF and their variances, and provides the corresponding plot. The variance of the CIF is estimated based on the delta method. The macro gives only the estimates and the graphs for the event of interest chosen by the user. The estimates for the conditional probability, discussed in Chapter 8, are also calculated.

The use of the `cuminc` macro is illustrated on the bone marrow transplant dataset. Suppose that the latter is already in a SAS dataset format named `bmt`. As before, one has to create the time variable which represents the earliest time when an event occurred and the censoring variable. For the latter the same codes are preserved: 0 if no event was observed, 1 for CGVHD, 2 for relapse and 3 for death:

```
data bmt;
set bmt;
earliest = min(cgvhtime,reltime,survtime);
event = (earliest=cgvhtime and cgvh=1)+
      2*(earliest=reltime and rcens=1)+
      3*(earliest=survtime and stat=1);
run;
```

The parameters for the macro `cuminc` are the name of the dataset (`ds=`), the name of the time variable (`time=`), the name of the event type variable (`cenvble=`), the numeric code for the event type of interest (`interest=`), and the name of the grouping variable (`group=`). For our example the statement is:

```
%cuminc(ds=bmt,time=earliest,cenvble=event, interest=1,
  group=tx)
```

Since the results are the same as shown earlier, the output and plots are omitted.

4.4 CLOSING REMARKS

This chapter has presented a method for summarizing and graphically displaying time-to-event data that arise within a competing risks framework. During the past decade, the use of CIF has slowly replaced the straightforward Kaplan–Meier estimator when competing risks are present. Different authors have approached the estimation of CIF and its confidence intervals from different angles. Matthews (1988) derived the confidence intervals using the likelihood-based method. Dinse and Larson (1986) used a semi-Markov model and obtained the same estimator for the variance as that based on the delta method. The performance of the Dinse and Larson method is discussed in detail by Choudhury (2002). Pepe and Fleming (1991) and Lin (1997) developed other variance estimators using a counting process martingale formulation. In this chapter Aalen's (1978a) estimate and the delta method have been discussed; the former is used in the `cmprsk` package and the derivation of the latter is relatively easy to follow. The next chapter presents techniques for comparing two or more groups with respect to their CIFs or hazards of the CIFs.

5

Testing a covariate

5.1 INTRODUCTION

An important question in some statistical analyses is whether one group fares better than another group with respect to the outcome. Chapter 2 gave a brief presentation of methods to address this issue when the outcome is the time to the event in the absence of competing risks. This chapter is concerned with answering this question when competing risks are present. Note that the *cause-specific hazard* is the hazard of the marginal distribution as defined in ((3.7)) and the *hazard of the subdistribution* is the hazard defined by Gray (1988),

$$\gamma(t) = \frac{f(t)}{1 - F(t)},\tag{5.1}$$

where f is the subdensity for the event of interest and F is the subdistribution function for the event of interest. The hazard of the subdistribution can be interpreted as the probability of observing an event of interest in the next time interval while knowing that either the event of interest did not happen until then or that the competing risks event was observed. Depending on the clinical or medical question we want to answer, we may want to compare the cause-specific hazard or the cumulative incidence functions.

Competing Risks: A Practical Perspective   M. Pintilie
© 2006 John Wiley & Sons, Ltd

In the absence of competing risks the survivor function is a monotonic function of the hazard; in the presence of competing risks this property does not hold. Gray (1988) showed that there are situations when the cause-specific hazard in one group is larger than in the other group, while in terms of the cumulative incidence functions the inequality may change direction at a certain point in time. Figure 5.1 gives such an example. The two curves represent the CIFs for two groups. The time to the event of interest follows an exponential distribution with hazards $\lambda_{ev1} = 0.1$ for group 1 and $\lambda_{ev2} = 0.2$ for group 2. The times to the competing risk events for the two groups follow exponential distributions with hazards $\lambda_{cr1} = 0.1$ and $\lambda_{cr2} = 0.4$ for group 1 and group 2, respectively. It is assumed that the time to the event of interest is independent of the time to the competing risk events. Although the cause-specific hazard for group 2 is higher than for group 1 ($\lambda_{ev2} > \lambda_{ev1}$) the CIF for group 2 drops below the curve for group 1 at about 5 years. This is caused by the dependency of the CIF, not only on the cause-specific hazard of the event of interest, but also on the cause-specific hazard for the competing risk. In this way the question of what to compare becomes essential.

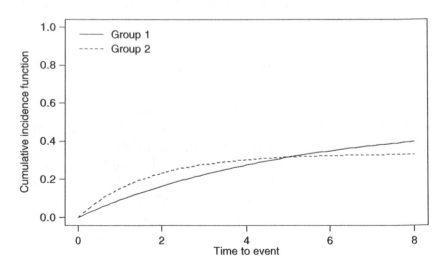

Figure 5.1 Non-monotonic relationship between cause-specific hazard and CIF.

The comparison of the cause-specific hazards is made as if the other types of events did not exist. Although this approach may seem unrealistic at first sight, it is a good way of analysing the data when one wants to find the biological mechanism underlying the specific outcome. On the other hand, comparing the CIFs is more direct, it takes into account all types of events and does not assume independence between the time to the different types of events. However, the CIF for the event of interest can be low just because the risk of a competing risk event is high. Hence, the simple comparison of the CIF for the event of interest is not sufficient and needs to be enhanced by the comparison of the CIF for the competing risks as well. An overview of advantages for each of these approaches is given in Table 5.1.

The example given in Chapter 1 regarding the comparison between the young an old groups of Hodgkin's disease patients (Figure 1.3) provides one instance where the test based on the cause-specific hazard (log-rank test) gives dramatically different results from the test based on the hazard of the subdistribution (Gray's test). As discussed, the two analyses actually complement each other. The log-rank test suggests that the older group has a higher risk of second malignancy, if the other risks are ignored. On the other hand, Gray's test on the event of interest (second malignancy) as well as on the competing risk (death without second malignancy) indicates that due to other fatal conditions the older

Table 5.1 Advantages of the two main approaches to analysing data in the presence of the competing risks.

Comparing the CIF or its hazard	Comparing the cause-specific hazard
It is a direct approach. It compares the observed probabilities of events or the observed rates of events.	It gives insight into the biological mechanism.
It does not assume independence between the types of events.	It is invariant to the size of the competing risks.
Some software has recently been made available.	The software is available in most statistical packages.

group experiences about the same number of second malignancies as the younger group.

In general, comparing the cause-specific hazards gives an insight into the biological process, while comparing the CIFs gives an idea of the probability of failure and therefore can be translated into actual numbers of patients with failure. Gray (1988) notes that the monotonic relationship between the cause-specific hazard and the CIF is preserved if the distribution of the time to the first failure of any type is the same in the groups that are compared.

To compare the cause-specific hazards one can apply the usual survival techniques available in the common statistical software programs such as the log-rank test and the Cox proportional hazards model (Pintilie, 2002). However, special techniques are needed to compare the cumulative incidence functions or the hazard of the subdistributions. In the next section we present two tests: Gray's test based on the hazard of the subdistribution and the test introduced by Pepe and Mori (1993) which compares two CIFs.

5.2   TESTING A COVARIATE

5.2.1   Gray's method

Without loss of generality, only two types of events are considered: the event of interest and the competing risk event. Since the functions involved in the test refer to the event of interest, the index for the type of event is suppressed.

The k-sample test introduced by Gray (1988) compares the weighted averages of the hazard of the subdistribution functions for the event of interest. The general form of the score for group i is

$$z_i = \int_0^\tau W_i(t) \left\{ \gamma_i(t) - \gamma_0(t) \right\} dt, \tag{5.2}$$

where τ is the maximum time observed in both groups, $W_i(t)$ is a weight function, $\gamma_i(t)$ is the hazard of the subdistribution for group i defined in (5.1) and $\gamma_0(t)$ is the hazard of the subdistribution for all groups together. In general, the weight function is of the form $W_i(t) = L(t) R_i(t)$ for some function $L(t)$ and

$$R_i(t) = n_i(t) \frac{1 - \hat{F}_i(t-)}{\hat{S}_i(t-)}, \tag{5.3}$$

where $n_i(t)$ is number of individuals at risk at time t in group i, $F(t-)$ is the left-hand limit of the CIF for the event of interest and $S(t-)$ is the left-hand limit of the probability of being free of any event, as estimated by the Kaplan–Meier method. In this way, R_i represents an adjusted number of individuals at risk.

It may be observed that $\sum z_k = 0$. The test statistic is a quadratic form using Z and the variance–covariance matrix. Under the null hypothesis this test statistic is distributed as χ^2_{k-1}.

For the sake of clarity, this test is presented for $k = 2$ and $L(t) = 1$ in the discrete case. It is obvious that only z_1 needs to be calculated and that $W_1(t) = R_1(t)$. Let $t_1, t_2, \ldots, t_n$ be the ordered time points when an event of any kind in any group occurred, d_{1j} the number of events of interest in group 1 at time t_j and n_{1j} the number at risk in group 1 at time t_j. Then

$$R_{1j} = n_{1j} \frac{1 - \hat{F}_1(t_{j-1})}{\hat{S}_1(t_{j-1})} \tag{5.4}$$

and the score is

$$\begin{aligned} Z_1 &= \sum_{\text{all } t_j} W(t_j) \left(\frac{d_{1j}}{R_{1j}} - \frac{d_{1j} + d_{2j}}{R_{1j} + R_{2j}} \right) \\ &= \sum_{\text{all } t_j} R_{1j} \left(\frac{d_{1j}}{R_{1j}} - \frac{d_{1j} + d_{2j}}{R_{1j} + R_{2j}} \right). \end{aligned} \tag{5.5}$$

Formula (5.5) closely resembles the form of the log-rank test (formula (2.11)) if the R_{1j} are interpreted as the modified number at risk. Note that z_1 is only the numerator of the statistic used in this test. The formula for the variance, which represents the denominator of the test statistic, is cumbersome (but see Appendix A). Table 5.2 shows the calculations for the score for a hypothetical example comparing the hazard of the subdistribution for type 1 event between group A and group B.

Table 5.2 Example for the calculation of the numerator of Gray's test.

Time	Event	Group	n_A	n_B	F_A	F_B	S_A	S_B	R_A	R_B	Terms for z_A
1	2	B	13	7	0	0	1	0.85714	13	7	0
2	2	A	13	6	0	0	0.92308	0.85714	13	7	0
3	0	A	12	6	0	0	0.92308	0.85714	13	7	0
4	1	B	11	6	0	0.14286	0.92308	0.71429	11.9167	7	−0.63
5	1	A	11	5	0.08392	0.14286	0.83916	0.71429	11.9167	6	0.335
6	0	A	10	5	0.08392	0.14286	0.83916	0.71429	10.9167	6	0
7	2	B	9	5	0.08392	0.14286	0.83916	0.57143	9.825	6	0
8	0	A	9	4	0.08392	0.14286	0.83916	0.57143	9.825	6	0
9	1	B	8	4	0.08392	0.28571	0.83916	0.42857	8.7333	6	−0.593
10	0	A	8	3	0.08392	0.28571	0.83916	0.42857	8.7333	5	0
11	2	A	7	3	0.08392	0.28571	0.71928	0.42857	7.6417	5	0
12	1	A	6	3	0.2038	0.28571	0.5994	0.42857	7.6417	5	0.396
13	1	A	5	3	0.32368	0.28571	0.47952	0.42857	6.6417	5	0.429
14	2	A	4	3	0.32368	0.28571	0.35964	0.42857	5.6417	5	0
15	2	B	3	3	0.32368	0.28571	0.35964	0.28571	5.6417	5	0
16	1	A	3	2	0.44356	0.28571	0.23976	0.28571	5.6417	5	0.47
17	1	B	2	2	0.44356	0.42857	0.23976	0.14286	4.6417	5	−0.481
18	1	A	2	1	0.56344	0.42857	0.11988	0.14286	4.6417	4	0.463
											$Z = 0.388$

A,B = indices for the groups; n = number at risk; F = CIF; S = probability of being free of any event; R = modified number at risk.

5.2.2 Pepe and Mori's method

Pepe and Mori (1993) give a method for comparing the cumulative incidence curves directly. This test is based on Pepe's earlier work (Pepe, 1991) where the author gave a test for comparing two survivor functions. We observe here that what they call 'marginal' is different than the notion presented in Chapter 3 of this book. The test is essentially the weighted area between the two CIFs.

It was proven by Pepe (1991) that under the null hypothesis

$$s = \sqrt{\frac{N_1 N_2}{N_1 + N_2}} \int_0^\tau W(t) \{F_1(t) - F_2(t)\} \, dt$$

is asymptotically normal with mean 0 and standard deviation σ. In this formula $F_i(t)$ represents the cumulative incidence function for the event of interest for group i, N_i is the total number of subjects in group i and $W(t)$ is a weight function. For the discrete case where $t_1, t_2, \ldots, t_n$ are the ordered unique time points for all observations (events or not) in both groups, the above formula becomes

$$s = \sqrt{\frac{N_1 N_2}{N_1 + N_2}} \sum_{\text{all } t_j} \left\{ W(t_j) \left[\hat{F}_1(t_j) - \hat{F}_2(t_j) \right] (t_{j+1} - t_j) \right\}. \tag{5.6}$$

The weight function is given by

$$W(t_j) = \frac{(N_1 + N_2) \, \hat{C}_1(t_{j-1}) \, \hat{C}_2(t_{j-1})}{N_1 \hat{C}_1(t_{j-1}) + N_2 \hat{C}_2(t_{j-1})} \tag{5.7}$$

where $1 - \hat{C}(t)$ is the Kaplan–Meier estimator of the censoring distribution. Note that $C(t)$ is the Kaplan–Meier estimator of the survivor function where the events are defined as the observations which are either censored or competing risks events. This means that formula (5.6) changes every time an event of interest occurs (due to changes in the CIF) but also when at the previous time point the observation has either been censored or a competing risk has occurred (due to changes in $C(t)$). The weight function is a decreasing function of time, therefore its effect on s is to give less weight to the difference in the CIFs as the time increases. This is intuitively appealing since it is known that the number of observations still in the risk set decreases as the time progresses. Table 5.3 illustrates the calculation of s on a hypothetical example comparing the CIF for a type 1 event between group A and group B. The shaded region in Figure 5.2 is the weighted area calculated for this test.

The variance of s is estimated as the weighted average of the variances of the two groups:

$$\hat{\sigma}^2 = \frac{N_1 N_2 \left(\hat{\sigma}_1^2 + \hat{\sigma}_2^2\right)}{N_1 + N_2}.$$

Table 5.3 Example for the calculation of the test for CIF introduced by Pepe and Mori.

Time	Events	Group	F_A	F_B	W	$W\left(F_A - F_B\right)\left(t_{j+1} - t_j\right)$
1	2	B	0.0000	0.0000	1.0000	0.0000
2	2	A	0.0000	0.0000	0.9023	0.0000
3	0	A	0.0000	0.0000	0.8791	0.0000
4	1	B	0.0000	0.1429	0.8533	−0.1219
5	1	A	0.0839	0.1429	0.8533	−0.0503
6	0	A	0.0839	0.1429	0.8533	−0.0503
7	2	B	0.0839	0.1429	0.8211	−0.0484
8	0	A	0.0839	0.1429	0.7105	−0.0419
9	1	B	0.0839	0.2857	0.6826	−0.1377
10	0	A	0.0839	0.2857	0.6826	−0.1377
11	2	A	0.0839	0.2857	0.6498	−0.1311
12	1	A	0.2038	0.2857	0.6108	−0.0500
13	1	A	0.3237	0.2857	0.6108	0.0232
14	2	A	0.3237	0.2857	0.6108	0.0232
15	2	B	0.3237	0.2857	0.5356	0.0203
16	1	A	0.4436	0.2857	0.4272	0.0674
17	1	B	0.4436	0.4286	0.4272	0.0064
18	1	A	0.5634	0.4286	0.4272	0.0576
19	0	A	–	–	–	–
20	0	B	–	–	–	–
						Total $= -0.5713$
						$s = -1.2186$

A,B $=$ indices for the groups; $F =$ CIF; $W =$ weight calculated based on (5.7); $N_A = 13, N_B = 7$.

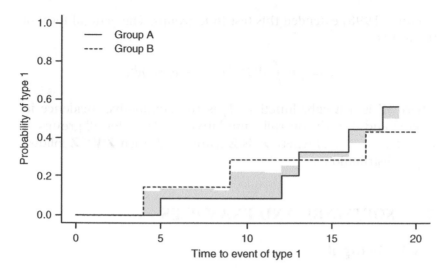

Figure 5.2 Illustration of the weighted area between the two curves calculated using the method of Pepe and Mori.

Since the calculation of the variance is the same in each of the two groups the estimator for only one group is given and the index i for the group is suppressed. In this way n_j is the number at risk at time t_j in group i, d_j is the number of events (of interest or competing risk) at time t_j in group i and d_{evj} refers to the number of events of interest at time t_j in group i. In the same way F is really the CIF for the event of interest for group i, F_{cr} is the CIF for the competing risk for group i and σ is the standard deviation for group i. The formula for the variance for group i is

$$\hat{\sigma}^2 = \sum_{\text{all } t_j} \frac{\left[v_1\left(t_j\right) - \hat{F}_{cr}\left(t_j\right) v_2\left(t_j\right)\right]^2 d_{evj} + v_2^2\left(t_j\right)\left(d_j - d_{evj}\right)}{n_j\left(n_j - 1\right)},$$

where

$$v_1\left(t_j\right) = \sum_{t_k \geq t_j} W\left(t_k\right)\left(t_{k+1} - t_k\right)\left(1 - \hat{F}\left(t_k\right)\right),$$

$$v_2\left(t_j\right) = \sum_{t_k \geq t_j} W\left(t_k\right)\left(t_{k+1} - t_k\right).$$

Lunn (1998) extended this test to k groups. The general form of the test is

$$z_i = \sqrt{n_i} \int W(t) \{F_i(t) - F_0(t)\} dt,$$

where W is a weight function, F_i is the cumulative incidence in group i and F_0 is the overall cumulative incidence for all groups. If $\mathbf{Z}^t = (z_1, z_2, \ldots, z_k,)$ where $\mathbf{Z}^t$ is $\mathbf{Z}$ transposed, then $\mathbf{Z}^t \mathbf{V}^{-1} \mathbf{Z}$ follows a χ^2_{k-1} distribution.

5.3   SOFTWARE AND EXAMPLES

5.3.1   Using R

The use of the log-rank test, Gray's test and the test introduced by Pepe and Mori are exemplified using the Follicular cell lymphoma dataset (`follic`, see Chapter 1). The event of interest is failure from the disease: either no response to treatment or relapse. Death without failure constitutes a competing risk type of event. There are 272 events of interest (24 non-responders, 248 relapses) and 76 observations experiencing the competing risk event (death without relapse). Two groups are defined based on age, dichotomized at 65.

It is assumed that the `cmprsk` library, which also contains the `survival` library, has already been loaded (see Section 4.3.1) and that the data have been imported (as shown in Appendix B). The variable that we want to test can be created as follows:

```
>a=(follic$age>65)+0
```

Adding the zero creates a numeric object (values 1 for TRUE and 0 for FALSE) rather than an object of type 'logical' (values TRUE or FALSE).

The next step is to create the indicator variables for the event of interest and for the competing risks. We create `evcens`, the indicator variable for the event of interest, which takes the value 1 if either there is no response or there is a relapse and 0 otherwise. Similarly, the indicator variable for the competing risks, `crcens`, is created:

```
>evcens=(follic$resp=='NR' | follic$relsite!='')+0
>crcens=(follic$resp=='CR' & follic$relsite=='' &
follic$stat==1)+0
```

The time to event is **dftime**. The cause-specific hazards are compared using the function **survdiff** which gives the value of the chi-square statistic with one degree of freedom ($k = 2$). The *p*-value can be found using the following commands:

```
> fit=survdiff(Surv(follic$dftime,evcens) ~ a)
> fit$chisq
[1] 6.941658
> lrpvalue=1-pchisq(fit$chisq,1)
> lrpvalue
[1] 0.008421103
```

The *p*-value based on Gray's test is calculated using the function **cuminc**. We create first the censoring variable, which needs to be coded as 1 for the event of interest and 2 for the competing risk.

```
>cens=evcens+2*crcens
```

The function can now be applied:

```
>fit=cuminc(follic$dftime,cens,a,cencode=0)
```

If the coding for the censored value is different, it can be specified using the parameter **cencode**. By typing **fit** we obtain the results of the Gray's test for both endpoints: the event of interest on the first line, marked with '1', and the test for the competing risks, marked with '2', reflecting the way the **cens** variable was coded.

```
> fit
Tests:
          stat            pv    df
1      2.631747   1.047464e-01    1
2     39.309879   3.616071e-10    1
Estimates and Variances:
```

```
$est              5            10            15            20          25          30
0 1    0.35195419    0.47049030    0.52699947    0.5548075   0.5676301   0.5676301
1 1    0.43918702    0.54144791    0.57190811    0.5719081          NA          NA
0 2    0.02631277    0.04830215    0.08347274    0.1246275   0.1562566   0.3257820
1 2    0.11606747    0.21218284    0.30365127    0.3285394          NA          NA

$var              5            10            15            20            25            30
0 1  0.0006021053  0.0007310347  0.0008054858  0.0009009575  0.001012861  0.001012861
1 1  0.0015928084  0.0017991588  0.0018575745  0.0018575745           NA           NA
0 2  0.0000676681  0.0001330323  0.0002740211  0.0005138645  0.000943020  0.012360082
1 2  0.0006696585  0.0012829053  0.0018782212  0.0023042993           NA           NA
```

In this case the *p*-value obtained ($p = 0.105$) is clearly different than that obtained using the log-rank test ($p = 0.008$), suggesting that the competing risks are quite different between these two groups. This fact is supported by the *p*-value for the competing risk found on the second line ($p < 0.0001$).

As shown in Chapter 4, we can plot each of these curves (Figure 5.3) using the following commands:

```
> forplev=list(list(fit$'0 1'$time,fit$'0 1'$est),
    list(fit$'1 1'$time,fit$'1 1'$est))

> plot.cuminc(forplev,curvlab=c('Age<=65','Age>65'),lty=c(1,2),
    xlab='Time to disease failure (years)',
    ylab='Probability for disease failure')
> title(main='Follicular dataset: CIFs for disease failure')
```

The *p*-values can be written on the graph as follows:

```
> text(0,0.75,adj=0,paste("Log-rank test: p-value=",
              round(lrpvalue,3)))
> text(0,0.8,adj=0,paste("Gray's test: p-value=",
              round(fit$Tests[1,2],3)))
```

The curves for the competing risk can be drawn as already shown (Figure 5.4):

```
> forplcr=list(list(fit$'0 2'$time,fit$'0 2'$est),
                list(fit$'1
2'$time,fit$'12'$est))
> plot.cuminc(forplcr,curvlab=c('Age<=65','Age>65'), lty=c(1,2),
    xlab='Time to death without disease failure (years)',
    ylab='Probability for competing risk')
> title(main='Follicular dataset: CIFs for competing risk')
> text(0,0.8,adj=0,paste("Gray's test: p-value=",
        round(fit$Tests[2,2],3)))
```

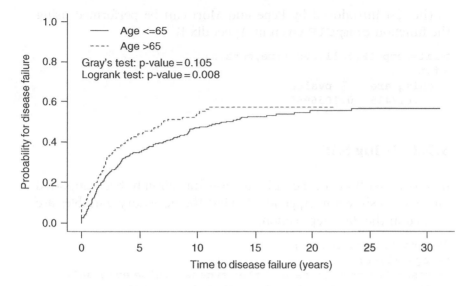

Figure 5.3 CIFs for disease failure.

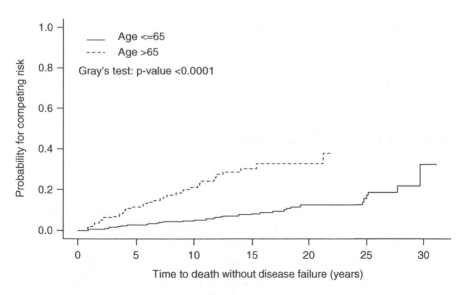

Figure 5.4 CIFs for competing risk.

The test introduced by Pepe and Mori can be performed using the function `compCIF` given in Appendix B:

```
> fit=compCIF(follic$dftime,cens,a)
> fit
  chisquare       pvalue
  2.617415   0.1056965
```

5.3.2   Using SAS

It is assumed that the `follic` dataset has already been imported into SAS as shown in Appendix B. First the necessary variables are created in the datastep section.

```
data follic;set follic;
a=(age>65)+0;
if resp='NR' or relsite^=' ' then evcens=1;else evcens=0;
if resp='CR' and relsite=' ' and stat=1 then crcens=1;
  else crcens=0;
cens=evcens+2*crcens;
```

The log-rank test can be applied using `proc lifetest`.

```
proc lifetest data=follic;
time dftime*evcens(0);strata a;
```

To perform the test introduced by Pepe and Mori, use the macro `compcif`:

```
%compcif(ds=follic, time=dftime, cens=cens,group=a, val1=0,
  val2=1)
```

5.4   CLOSING REMARKS

This chapter has presented two fundamentally different approaches to testing a covariate in the presence of competing risks. If the goal is to examine the biological effect of the covariate, we have to test the cause-specific hazard. In this case the usual survival techniques available in the established statistical software (such as the log-rank test or the Cox proportional hazards model) can be used. On the other hand, if the goal is to assess whether there are differences between proportions of patients experiencing a certain condition in time then we have to compare the CIFs. When cause-specific hazards are compared competing risk are ignored, and therefore the results change only if the risk for the event of interest changes. Comparing the CIFs or their hazards takes into account the competing risks. Thus, the difference between the CIFs may appear larger (or smaller) in a population just because the competing risks are different. Therefore, an analysis of the CIFs for the event of interest needs to be accompanied by some information on the competing risks.

Although there are other methods in the literature for testing a covariate in the presence of competing risks, only those introduced by Gray and by Pepe and Mori have been presented here. Both can be applied readily since Gray's method is implemented in R, while for Pepe and Mori's method an R function as well as an SAS macro have been written (Appendix B). In this chapter these tests have been applied to a real-life example.

Other tests for comparing two groups while adjusting for the competing risks have been developed. A rank-type test was given by Lin *et al.* (1996). Lin (1997) proposed an omnibus-type test. Kulathinal and Gasbarra (2002) introduced a test for comparing the cause-specific cumulative hazard function, which can give an overall significance for K groups and m types of events without assuming independence between the different types of events.

Modelling in the presence of competing risks

6.1 INTRODUCTION

The previous chapters have discussed the two possible approaches to testing a covariate: testing the cause-specific hazard and testing the hazard of the subdistribution. The present chapter examines how each of these hazards can be modelled. The avenue taken depends on the medical question of interest.

6.2 MODELLING THE HAZARD OF THE CUMULATIVE INCIDENCE FUNCTION

6.2.1 Theoretical details

This section presents the work of Fine and Gray (1999) on modelling the hazard of the CIF. The methodology has many points in common with both the k-sample test introduced by Gray (1988) and the Cox proportional hazards model (see Section 2.3.3). Although the theory is developed gradually (starting with the case of no censoring), the general case for incomplete data is presented here. This is the type of data which we usually encounter: there are individuals with an event of interest recorded, others with a

Competing Risks: A Practical Perspective M. Pintilie
© 2006 John Wiley & Sons, Ltd

competing risk type of event and yet others who are censored. The model is based on

$$\gamma(t, \mathbf{x}) = \gamma_0(t) e^{\beta \mathbf{x}},$$

where γ is the hazard of the subdistribution, γ_0 is the baseline hazard of the subdistribution, $\mathbf{x}$ is the vector of the covariates and $\boldsymbol{\beta}$ is the vector of the coefficients.

The form of the partial likelihood is similar to that used in the Cox proportional hazards model (2.16). Written for just one covariate, x, the partial likelihood is given by the formula

$$L(\beta) = \prod_{j=1}^{r} \frac{\exp(\beta x_j)}{\sum_{i \in R_j} w_{ji} \exp(\beta x_i)}. \tag{6.1}$$

The product is taken over r all time points $(t_1 < t_2 < \ldots < t_r)$, where an event of interest was observed. There are two main differences between (6.1) and (2.16). The risk set R_j is defined in a different way and weights w_{ji} are added. The risk set is formed of those who did not experience an event by time t and of those who experienced a competing risk event by time t:

$$R_j(t) = \{i;\ T_i \geq t \quad \text{or} \quad (T_i \leq t \text{ and the subject experienced a competing risk event})\}. \tag{6.2}$$

Thus, those who experienced other types of events remain in the risk set all the time. The weights are defined as

$$w_{ji} = \frac{\hat{G}(t_j)}{\hat{G}(\min(t_j, t_i))}, \tag{6.3}$$

where $\hat{G}$ is the Kaplan–Meier estimate of the survivor function of the censoring distribution. The censoring distribution is defined by (T_i, C_i), where T_i is the time to the first event and C_i is 1 if no event was observed and 0 if any kind of event was observed. At each time point where an event of interest occurred (indexed by j) the set of individuals at risk (indexed by i) includes those who did not have any type of event by time t_j as well as those who had a competing risks event before t_j. The weight is 1 for the former and less than or equal to 1 for the latter. In this way those individuals experiencing a competing risk event do not participate fully in the partial likelihood: the further the time point (t_j) is from the time when the competing risk event occurred, the smaller the weight.

Applying the derivative to the log of the partial likelihood given in (6.1) gives the score statistic, which has the form

$$U(\beta) = \sum_{j=1}^{r} \left\{ x_j - \frac{\sum_{i \in R_j} w_{ji} x_i \exp(x_i \beta)}{\sum_{i \in R_j} w_{ji} \exp(x_i \beta)} \right\}. \tag{6.4}$$

The estimate of β, denoted by $\hat{\beta}$, is the value which maximizes the function $U(\beta)$. $\hat{\beta}$ does not have a closed form. Equation (6.4) can be written for a set of covariates and can be extended to include time-dependent covariates.

For the sake of clarity, the form of the score statistic is given for a simple example with only a few events of interest. When the number of events of interest is large the expression for the score statistic becomes cumbersome and its maximization is an elaborate task. Table 6.1 gives the data points as well as the estimates for $\hat{G}$.

Table 6.1 Hypothetical example dataset.

Individual	Time	Type of event	X	$\hat{G}$
SN1	1	0	12	0.9
SN2	2	2	10	0.9
SN3	3	1	9	0.9
SN4	4	1	13	0.9
SN5	5	0	8	0.75
SN6	6	2	9	0.75
SN7	7	1	12	0.75
SN8	8	0	10	0.5
SN9	9	1	11	0.5
SN10	10	0	8	0

X = covariate; $\hat{G}$ = estimator of the censoring distribution.
Type of event: 1 = Event of interest, 2 = Competing risk event, 0 = Censored.

Since there are only four events of interest (type 1), the score statistic has four terms. Note that for each time t_j the only weights other than 1 are those for previous time points t_i, $t_i < t_j$. The weights calculated for t_i, $t_i \geq t_j$, are 1 because $\min(t_j, t_i) = t_j$ and formula (6.3) becomes

$$w_{ji} = \frac{\hat{G}(t_j)}{\hat{G}(\min(t_j, t_i))} = \frac{\hat{G}(t_j)}{\hat{G}(t_j)} = 1.$$

Table 6.2 contains the values for the weights. The rows represent the four failure time points. For each of these events times the weights are calculated for each observation in the risk set, where the risk set is defined as in (6.2). The shaded cells correspond to the observations that are not in the risk set at that time point.

The events of interest were observed at $t = 3, 4, 7$ and 9. Hence the table has only 4 rows. Individual SN1 was censored at time $t = 1$, before any events of interest occurred. He is never in the risk set and he does not participate in the partial likelihood. Individual SN2 had a competing risk event at time $t = 2$. He is always in the risk set but with weight decreasing as time passes (from 1 to 0.56). Individual SN3 has an event of interest at time $t = 3$ and participates in the partial likelihood just for the first term with a weight of 1.

Table 6.2 Calculation of the weights for example in Table 6.1.

Time	SN1	SN2	SN3	SN4	SN5	SN6	SN7	SN8	SN9	SN10
3		$\dfrac{\hat{G}(3)}{\hat{G}(2)} = 1$	1	1	1	1	1	1	1	1
4		$\dfrac{\hat{G}(4)}{\hat{G}(2)} = 1$		1	1	1	1	1	1	1
7		$\dfrac{\hat{G}(7)}{\hat{G}(2)} = 0.83$				$\dfrac{\hat{G}(7)}{\hat{G}(6)} = 1$	1	1	1	1
9		$\dfrac{\hat{G}(9)}{\hat{G}(2)} = 0.56$				$\dfrac{\hat{G}(9)}{\hat{G}(6)} = 0.67$			1	1

For this example the score statistic, which needs to be maximized, is:

$$U(\beta) = x_3 - \frac{w_{32}x_2\exp(x_2\beta) + w_{33}x_3\exp(x_3\beta) + w_{34}x_4\exp(x_4\beta) + \ldots + w_{3,10}x_{10}\exp(x_{10}\beta)}{w_{32}\exp(x_2\beta) + w_{33}\exp(x_3\beta) + w_{34}\exp(x_4\beta) + \ldots + w_{3,10}\exp(x_{10}\beta)}$$

$$+ x_4 - \frac{w_{42}x_2\exp(x_2\beta) + w_{44}x_4\exp(x_4\beta) + w_{45}x_5\exp(x_5\beta) + \ldots + w_{4,10}x_{10}\exp(x_{10}\beta)}{w_{42}\exp(x_2\beta) + w_{44}\exp(x_4\beta) + w_{45}\exp(x_5\beta) + \ldots + w_{4,10}\exp(x_{10}\beta)}$$

$$+ x_7 - \frac{w_{72}x_2\exp(x_2\beta) + w_{76}x_6\exp(x_6\beta) + w_{77}x_7\exp(x_7\beta) + \ldots + w_{7,10}x_{10}\exp(x_{10}\beta)}{w_{72}\exp(x_2\beta) + w_{76}\exp(x_6\beta) + w_{77}\exp(x_7\beta) + \ldots + w_{7,10}\exp(x_{10}\beta)}$$

$$+ x_9 - \frac{w_{92}x_2\exp(x_2\beta) + w_{96}x_6\exp(x_6\beta) + w_{99}x_9\exp(x_9\beta) + w_{9,10}x_{10}\exp(x_{10}\beta)}{w_{92}\exp(x_2\beta) + w_{96}\exp(x_6\beta) + w_{99}\exp(x_9\beta) + w_{9,10}\exp(x_{10}\beta)}.$$

Replacing the weight w_{ji} with the value found in row j and column i of Table 6.2 and substituting x with the value given in Table 6.1 gives:

$$U(\beta) = 9 - \frac{10e^{10\beta} + 9e^{9\beta} + 13e^{13\beta} + 8e^{8\beta} + 9e^{9\beta} + 12e^{12\beta} + 10e^{10\beta} + 11e^{11\beta} + 8e^{8\beta}}{e^{10\beta} + e^{9\beta} + e^{13\beta} + e^{8\beta} + e^{9\beta} + e^{12\beta} + e^{10\beta} + e^{11\beta} + e^{8\beta}}$$

$$+ 13 - \frac{10e^{10\beta} + 13e^{13\beta} + 8e^{8\beta} + 9e^{9\beta} + 12e^{12\beta} + 10e^{10\beta} + 11e^{11\beta} + 8e^{8\beta}}{e^{10\beta} + e^{13\beta} + e^{8\beta} + e^{9\beta} + e^{12\beta} + e^{10\beta} + e^{11\beta} + e^{8\beta}}$$

$$+ 12 - \frac{0.83 \times 10e^{10\beta} + 9e^{9\beta} + 12e^{12\beta} + 10e^{10\beta} + 11e^{11\beta} + 8e^{8\beta}}{0.83e^{10\beta} + e^{9\beta} + e^{12\beta} + e^{10\beta} + e^{11\beta} + e^{8\beta}}$$

$$+ 11 - \frac{0.56 \times 10e^{10\beta} + 0.67 \times 9e^{9\beta} + 11e^{11\beta} + 8e^{8\beta}}{0.56e^{10\beta} + 0.67e^{9\beta} + e^{11\beta} + e^{8\beta}}.$$

$$(6.5)$$

Using a computer (function `crr` in R), the maximum of this function is found to be at $\hat{\beta} = 0.666\,217$. Substituting this value in (6.5) gives, the value of the score statistic:

$$U\left(\hat{\beta}\right) = -2.774\,441\,5 + 1.137\,359\,0 + 0.983\,453\,9 + 0.653\,628\,6$$

$$= 8.9 \times 10^{-12}. \tag{6.6}$$

There are several points of interest. When there is only one type of event, the weights are all equal to 1 and the risk set contains only those individuals at risk at the specific time point. Therefore, the likelihood defined in (6.1) is identical to that for the Cox model. However, the covariance matrix is only asymptotically the same as in the Cox model. When there are complete data and the covariate is a dichotomous (0/1) variable, the score statistic defined in (6.4) is equivalent to that defined in (5.2) with weight $W = F_0/F_1F_2$, where F_0 stands for the cumulative incidence for the pooled data and F_1 and F_2 represent the cumulative incidence functions for group 1 and group 2, respectively. Based on simulations (Fine and Gray, 1999) for the incomplete data, the two score statistics are well correlated (with a correlation coefficient in excess of 0.97).

6.2.2 Model-based estimation of the CIF

The predicted CIF can be calculated for a certain value of the covariates using the formula

$$F(t) = 1 - \exp(-H(t)), \tag{6.7}$$

where $H(t)$ is the cumulative hazard of the subdistribution. $\hat{H}(t)$ can be calculated using a Breslow-type estimator:

$$\hat{H}\left(t; x_0, \hat{\beta}\right) = \sum_{t_j \leq t} \left\{ \frac{\exp\left(x_0 \hat{\beta}\right)}{\sum_{i \in R_j} w_{ji} \exp\left(x_i \hat{\beta}\right)} \right\}. \tag{6.8}$$

The outer sum is over all time points for which an event of interest was observed.

For the data in Table 6.1 the cumulative hazards calculated at $t = t_3$ and $t = t_9$ for $x_0 = 10$ and $\hat{\beta} = 0.666\,217$ are:

$$\hat{H}\left(t = 3; x_0 = 10, \hat{\beta}\right) = \frac{e^{10\hat{\beta}}}{e^{10\hat{\beta}} + e^{9\hat{\beta}} + e^{13\hat{\beta}} + e^{8\hat{\beta}} + e^{9\hat{\beta}} + e^{12\hat{\beta}} + e^{10\hat{\beta}} + e^{11\hat{\beta}} + e^{8\hat{\beta}}}$$

$$= 0.06$$

$$\hat{H}\left(t = 9; x_0 = 10, \hat{\beta}\right) = \frac{e^{10\hat{\beta}}}{e^{10\hat{\beta}} + e^{9\hat{\beta}} + e^{13\hat{\beta}} + e^{8\hat{\beta}} + e^{9\hat{\beta}} + e^{12\hat{\beta}} + e^{10\hat{\beta}} + e^{11\hat{\beta}} + e^{8\hat{\beta}}}$$

$$+ \frac{e^{10\hat{\beta}}}{e^{10\hat{\beta}} + e^{13\hat{\beta}} + e^{8\hat{\beta}} + e^{9\hat{\beta}} + e^{12\hat{\beta}} + e^{10\hat{\beta}} + e^{11\hat{\beta}} + e^{8\hat{\beta}}}$$

$$+ \frac{e^{10\hat{\beta}}}{0.83 e^{10\hat{\beta}} + e^{9\hat{\beta}} + e^{12\hat{\beta}} + e^{10\hat{\beta}} + e^{11\hat{\beta}} + e^{8\hat{\beta}}}$$

$$+ \frac{e^{10\hat{\beta}}}{0.56 e^{10\hat{\beta}} + 0.67 e^{9\hat{\beta}} + e^{11\hat{\beta}} + e^{8\hat{\beta}}}$$

$$= 0.06 + 0.062 + 0.12 + 0.322$$

$$= 0.564.$$

The estimates of the CIF are:

$$\hat{F}\left(t = 3; x_0 = 10, \hat{\beta}\right) = 1 - e^{-\hat{H}(3)} = 1 - e^{-0.06} = 0.058,$$

$$\hat{F}\left(t = 9; x_0 = 10, \hat{\beta}\right) = 1 - e^{-\hat{H}(9)} = 1 - e^{-0.564} = 0.431.$$

6.2.3   Using R

The function `crr` (competing risks regression), available in the `cmprsk` package (Appendix B), uses the regression model introduced in Section 6.2.1.

As an example, the dataset `hypox` described in Section 1.6.2 is analyzed. We are interested in whether the interstitial fluid pressure (IFP) has any influence on local relapse. Assume that the data have been imported into R and the `cmprsk` library has been loaded.

First the censoring variable is created:

```
> cens=(hypox$pelrec=='Y')+
       2*(hypox$disrec=='Y' & hypox$pelrec!='Y')
```

Note that the censoring variable is coded as 1 for the event of interest (local relapse with or without distant relapse) and as 2 for the competing risk event (distant relapse in the absence of local relapse). There are 33 events of interest and 17 observations for which competing risk was observed. In this dataset there are no deaths without relapse. The variable `dftime` represents the time to the first type of event, which in this case could be local relapse, distant relapse or both. The next step is to create the matrix of covariates:

```
> x=cbind(hypox$ifp,hypox$tumsize,(hypox$pelvicln!='Y')+0)
```

The last column of `x` is an indicator variable with the value 1 when the pelvic nodes were either negative or equivocal and 0 otherwise. We have now all the necessary elements to apply the `crr` function.

Let us first test whether IFP is significant by itself:

```
> fit=crr(hypox$dftime,cens,x[,1])
> fit
convergence: TRUE
coefficients:
[1] 0.03454
```

```
standard errors:
[1] 0.01707
two-sided p-values:
[1] 0.043
```

The result tells us first that convergence was reached and then it gives the coefficient, the standard error and the *p*-value. In this case IFP is marginally significant with a *p*-value of 0.043. The coefficient is positive which means that the higher values represent a higher risk for local relapse.

The next step is to test IFP when controlling for tumour size and nodal status, which are known clinical prognostic factors:

```
> fit=crr(hypox$dftime,cens,x)
> fit
convergence: TRUE
coefficients:
[1] 0.03267 0.26030 -0.77910
standard errors:
[1] 0.01724 0.09753 0.42780
two-sided p-values:
[1] 0.0580 0.0076 0.0690
```

The values of the coefficients, standard error and *p*-values are given in the same order as they appear in the matrix **x**. The p-value for IFP is 0.058, for tumour size it is 0.0076 and for nodal status it is 0.069. Thus, when the effect of IFP is adjusted for the two clinical factors, tumour size and nodal status, it becomes marginally non-significant. This analysis cannot be fully interpreted without examining the effect of these covariates on the competing risk.

The same model can be run for the competing risk (distant relapse only), by specifying that the code for the event of interest is 2:

```
> fit=crr(hypox$dftime,cens,x[,1],failcode=2)
> fit
convergence: TRUE
coefficients:
[1] 0.04307
standard errors:
[1] 0.02026
two-sided p-values:
[1] 0.034
```

For the competing risk the IFP, unadjusted, is found to be significant (*p*-value 0.034) and remains significant even in the full model (*p*-value 0.018):

```
> fit=crr(hypox$dftime,cens,x,failcode=2)
> fit
convergence: TRUE
coefficients:
[1] 0.05092 -0.15040 -0.18480
standard errors:
[1] 0.0216 0.1756 0.6608
two-sided p-values:
[1] 0.018 0.390 0.780
```

In conclusion, a local relapse for high IFP is less likely to be observed because it may be preceded by distant relapse. If the *p*-value for the analysis for local relapse (0.058) had been more convincingly non-significant it could have been suggested that there is no real need for new local treatment because the patients tend to relapse distantly first, therefore a systemic treatment would be more advantageous.

Some other elements of the modelling can be obtained. For example, the coefficients are given by

```
> fit$coef
[1] 0.05091501 -0.15042156 -0.18484486
```

and the covariance matrix of the coefficients is

```
> fit$var
              [,1]           [,2]           [,3]
[1,]    0.0004666954  -0.00169004   0.001877048
[2,]   -0.0016900398   0.03085194   0.023358791
[3,]    0.0018770482   0.02335879   0.436692221
```

Note that these last results do not express the association of IFP with distant relapse, but with competing risks for local relapse. In this dataset there are 15 events which are both local and distant and which are counted only towards the analysis for local relapse. Therefore, not all distant relapses are considered events in the competing risks analysis. The association between IFP and distant relapse (adjusted for the other parameters) produces the following results:

```
> cens=(hypox$disrec=='Y')+2*(hypox$disrec=='N' &
          hypox$pelrec=='Y')
> fit=crr(hypox$dftime,cens,x)
> fit
convergence: TRUE
coefficients:
[1] 0.03951 0.15580 -0.30030
standard errors:
[1] 0.01876 0.10910 0.47830
two-sided p-values:
[1] 0.035 0.150 0.530
```

Another output from the function crr is $res (fit$res for our example) which contains the components of the score statistics given by each covariate and each failure time point. Thus, fit$res is a matrix with as many columns as the number of covariates in the model and as many rows as the unique number of failure time points. For the hypothetical example in Section 6.2.1 the elements of fit$res are the terms of the sum in (6.6). For the last model presented (fit=crr(hypox$dftime,cens,x,failcode=2)) fit$res is:

```
> fit$res
```

	[,1]	[,2]	[,3]
[1,]	-12.09633848	-0.3601572	-0.8185251
[2,]	-3.18067376	4.6373318	-0.8242318
[3,]	-0.19728913	4.6615566	0.1714625
[4,]	17.90170775	-1.3147415	0.1723343
[5,]	-0.01586112	-1.3575166	0.1779412
[6,]	-14.11606490	-0.3749573	-0.8197727
[7,]	-0.38114830	0.6178886	0.1753770
[8,]	8.21517382	0.6238509	0.1770693
[9,]	5.25077024	0.6452314	0.1692324
[10,]	-9.67924536	-1.3461687	0.1714880
[11,]	3.03886073	-0.3575583	0.1729389
[12,]	0.08413954	-0.3354060	0.1766899
[13,]	9.78518777	-0.3395846	0.1788912
[14,]	-4.41088744	-0.3466616	0.1826193
[15,]	-3.55549230	-2.3501672	0.1844660
[16,]	-10.93029301	-1.3769660	0.1833147
[17,]	14.28745396	-1.3259743	0.1687048

The sum of each column is equal to the corresponding covariate score statistic:

```
> apply(fit$res,2,sum)
[1] 4.745315e-09 -1.669390e-09 6.980054e-10
> fit$score
[1] 4.745284e-09 -1.669394e-09 6.980047e-10
```

The function `predict.crr` computes the predicted CIF based on the model evaluated in `crr` as shown in formulae (6.7) and (6.8). The first input parameter of the function is an object, which is the output from the `crr` function. The second and third input parameters, `cov1` and `cov2`, are matrices of covariates and should have the same structure as their homologous parameters used in the call of the `crr` function. If one does not have time-dependent covariates (as in our example) then `cov2` is not used. Each row is a set of values of the covariates for which one wishes to calculate the predicted CIF. The result is a matrix with as many rows as the number of unique failure times. The number of columns is equal to the number of rows in `cov1` plus one for the time point. As an illustration let us calculate the estimate of CIF for local relapse, for the following four sets of data:

1. IFP = 5, tumour size= 5 and nodal status=negative/equivocal (value = 1),
2. IFP = 5, tumour size=5 and nodal status=positive (value = 0),
3. IFP = 20, tumour size=5 and nodal status=negative/equivocal (value = 1),
4. IFP = 20, tumour size=5 and nodal status=positive (value = 0).

First we set up the `cov1` matrix:

```
> px=matrix(c(5,5,1,5,5,0,20,5,1,20,5,0),ncol=3,byrow=T)
> px
      [,1]  [,2]  [,3]
[1,]     5     5     1
[2,]     5     5     0
[3,]    20     5     1
[4,]    20     5     0
```

Applying the function `predict.crr` gives:

```
> pfit=predict.crr(fit,px)
> pfit
```

```
           [,1]        [,2]        [,3]         [,4]        [,5]
[1,]      0.003  0.05034308  0.1064769   0.08085937   0.1678732
[2,]      0.706  0.05472090  0.1154301   0.08776561   0.1814403
[3,]      0.939  0.05913397  0.1244061   0.09470703   0.1949549
[4,]      0.991  0.06357419  0.1333873   0.10167039   0.2083900
[5,]      1.029  0.06802610  0.1423418   0.10863117   0.2216979
[6,]      1.073  0.07250123  0.1512924   0.11560710   0.2349124
[7,]      1.084  0.07712438  0.1604856   0.12279144   0.2483937
[8,]      1.112  0.08186003  0.1698464   0.13012705   0.2620252
[9,]      1.123  0.08670127  0.1793573   0.13760153   0.2757759
[10,]     1.246  0.09155461  0.1888324   0.14506958   0.2893752
[11,]     1.350  0.09643444  0.1982992   0.15255301   0.3028626
[12,]     1.530  0.10131940  0.2077157   0.16001875   0.3161789
[13,]     1.541  0.10621400  0.2170905   0.16747354   0.3293370
[14,]     1.741  0.11159663  0.2273304   0.17564187   0.3435959
[15,]     2.519  0.11707528  0.2376780   0.18392384   0.3578840
[16,]     2.606  0.12259742  0.2480314   0.19223873   0.3720579
[17,]     7.107  0.14908981  0.2966382   0.23166870   0.4369482
attr(,"class")
[1] "predict.crr"
```

The first column contains the unique failure time point and the following columns contain the CIF estimates based on the model for the data points given in 1–4. These results can be plotted using `plot.predict.crr` (Figure 6.1):

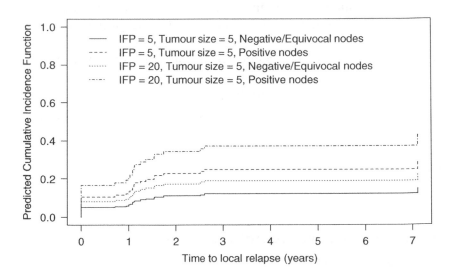

Figure 6.1 Predicted CIFs for four data points.

```
> par(las=1,mfrow=c(1,1))
> plot.predict.crr(pfit,lty=c(1:4),ylim=c(0,1),
  xlab='Time to local relapse',ylab='Predicted CIF')
> legend(0,1,lty=c(1:4),bty='n',
    legend=c('IFP=5, Tumour size=5, Negative/Equivocal nodes',
          'IFP=5, Tumour size=5, Postive nodes',
          'IFP=20, Tumour size=5, Negative/Equivocal nodes',
          'IFP=20, Tumour size=5, Postive nodes'))
```

Sometimes it is interesting to superimpose the CIF curve obtained from the observed data and the predicted CIF curve calculated using the model. The following statements create a plot of the observed and predicted CIF curves for positive nodes and negative/equivocal nodes (Figure 6.2):

```
> x=1-(hypox$pelvicln!='Y')+0
> fit=crr(hypox$dftime,cens,x)
> px=matrix(c(0,1),ncol=1)
> pfit=predict.crr(fit,px)
> par(las=1,mfrow=c(1,1))

> plot.predict.crr(pfit,lty=c(1:2),ylim=c(0,1),
    xlab='Time to local relapse',ylab='CIF')
> text(0,1,adj=0,'Predicted CIF',font=2)
> legend(0,1,lty=c(1:2),bty='n',
  legend=c('Negative/Equivocal nodes','Postive nodes'))
```

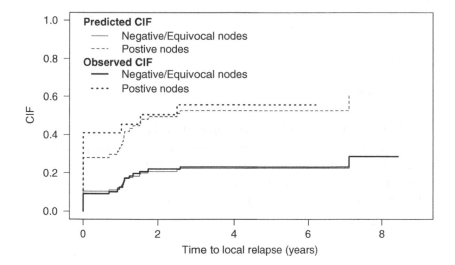

Figure 6.2 Observed and predicted CIFs.

```
> par(new=T)
> fitc=cuminc(hypox$dftime,cens,x)
> forplot=list(list(fitc$'0 1'$time,fitc$'0 1'$est),
               list(fitc$'1 1'$time,fitc$'1 1'$est))
> plot.cuminc(forplot,xlab='',ylab='',lty=c(1,3),lwd=2,
   wh=c(0,2))
> text(0,0.8,adj=0,'Observed CIF',font=2)
> legend(0,0.8,lty=c(1,3),bty='n',lwd=2,
     legend=c('Negative/Equivocal nodes','Postive nodes'))
```

The `crr` function can also accommodate time-dependent covariates, making it possible to model the hazard of subdistribution when the assumption of proportionality is not satisfied. As an example, let us test the variable `clinstg` (clinical stage) from the dataset `follic` introduced in Section 1.6.3. First, the association between the variable `clinstg` and the outcome (local relapse) is tested under the assumption of proportionality of hazards:

```
> evcens =(follic$resp=='NR' | follic$relsite!='')+0
> crcens=(follic$resp=='CR' & follic$relsite=='' &
    follic$stat==1)+0
> cens=evcens+2*crcens
```

The variable `clinstg` is recoded as 0 for clinical stage I and 1 for clinical stage II and renamed `stage`:

```
> stage=(follic$clinstg==2)+0
> fit=crr(follic$dftime,cens,stage)
> fit
convergence: TRUE
coefficients:
[1] 0.3748
standard errors:
[1] 0.127
two-sided p-values:
[1] 0.0032
```

Note that `stage` is significant (*p*-value 0.0032).

A linear interaction with time is considered first. The parameter `cov2` and the function that is applied to the variable `time` need to be supplied. In this case, cov2 is the covariate `stage`. The function is the identity and it is given by:

```
id=function(x)
{y=x
return(y)
}
```

The results obtained after applying the `crr` function are:

```
fittd=crr(follic$dftime,cens,stage,stage,id)
fittd
convergence: TRUE
coefficients:
[1] 0.69800 -0.09509
standard errors:
[1] 0.1662 0.0345
two-sided p-values:
[1] 2.7e-05 5.8e-03
```

Allowing the hazard ratio to change over time increases the coefficient for `stage` from 0.3748 to 0.698. The negative interaction coefficient (-0.09509) between time and clinical stage suggests that the hazard ratio is larger at the beginning and diminishes as time progresses. The first p-value (0.00003) shows that there is a significant increase in the hazard ratio between two groups at time 0. The second p-value (0.0058) indicates that the hazard ratio significantly decreases with time in a linear fashion.

In the next step a quadratic interaction term is introduced. The function used in `crr` for the parameter `tf` is created as follows:

```
idsq=function(x)
{
  y1=x
  y2=x*x
  y=cbind(y1,y2)
return(y)
}
```

Note that the parameter `cov2` needs to be a matrix of the same size as the return value of the function `idsq`.

```
> fitsq=crr(follic$dftime,cens,stage,cbind(stage,stage),idsq)
> fitsq
convergence: TRUE
coefficients:
[1] 0.672400 -0.077610 -0.001343
standard errors:
[1] 0.20520 0.07928 0.00457
two-sided p-values:
[1] 0.0011 0.3300 0.7700
```

The first p-value is for the variable `stage` at time 0, the second is for the interaction of `stage` with the time variable and the third is the interaction of `stage` with the square of the time variable. Both the coefficients and the p-values for the interaction terms suggest that the hazard ratio does not vary in a quadratic manner with time.

6.3   COX MODEL AND COMPETING RISKS

When the goal is to find the biological mechanism through which a specific characteristic influences the outcome, the cause-specific hazard must be modelled. Consider IFP from the `hypox` dataset and local relapse as the outcome. With the Fine and Gray model weak p-values for IFP were obtained (0.043 for the unadjusted analysis and 0.058 for the adjusted model). These results are influenced by the way the competing risks were distributed. If patients with high IFP were more likely to have a distant relapse the local relapse could not be observed and therefore the effect of IFP would be diminished. The reverse is true if the competing risks are more likely to happen in the low-IFP group. When the cause-specific hazard is modelled, the competing risks are ignored and thus the effect of the covariate reflects the 'pure' effect, when the other types of events do not exist. This is useful for formulating a new biological hypothesis. If the cause-specific hazard for local relapse increases with IFP, then the IFP is an important characteristic of tumour. Some questions may be derived: What causes the higher pressure in a tumour? How can it be lowered? Is this the main cause for the bad behaviour of tumours or is it a by-product of an underlining condition? Cause-specific hazards can be tested using Cox proportional hazards regression (`coxph` in R and `proc phreg` in SAS).

The IFP from the `hypox` dataset is tested alone in the model (unadjusted) as well as together with tumour size and nodal status (adjusted). The outcome is local relapse with the indicator variable `lcens`. It takes the value 1 when a local relapse was observed and 0 otherwise.

```
> fit=coxph(Surv(dftime,lcens)~ifp,data=hypox)
> fit
Call:
coxph(formula = Surv(dftime, lcens)~ifp, data = hypox)
```

```
          coef  exp(coef)  se(coef)      z      p
 ifp    0.0432       1.04    0.0187   2.31  0.021
```

```
Likelihood ratio test=4.97 on 1 df, p=0.0258 n= 109
> fit=coxph(Surv(dftime,lcens)~ifp+tumsize+(pelvicln=='Y'),
     data=hypox)
> fit
Call:
coxph(formula = Surv(dftime, lcens)~ifp + tumsize + (pelvicln
== "Y"), data = hypox)
```

```
                      coef  exp(coef)  se(coef)     z       p
ifp                 0.0425       1.04    0.0199  2.14  0.0320
tumsize             0.3110       1.36    0.0975  3.19  0.0014
pelvicln == "Y"TRUE 0.9579       2.61    0.4137  2.32  0.0210
```

```
Likelihood ratio test=28.0 on 3 df, p=3.7e-06 n= 109
```

Unlike the Fine and Gray method, the Cox regression found IFP significant in both models (unadjusted p-value=0.021 and adjusted p-value=0.032).

The same analysis is performed for distant relapse and IFP is again found to be significant:

```
> fit=coxph(Surv(dftime,dcens)~ifp,data=hypox)
> fit
Call:
coxph(formula = Surv(dftime, dcens) ~ ifp, data = hypox)
          coef  exp(coef)  se(coef)      z      p
ifp     0.0608       1.06    0.0189   3.21  0.0013
```

```
Likelihood ratio test=9.6 on 1 df, p=0.00194 n= 109
> fit=coxph(Surv(dftime,dcens)~ifp+tumsize+(pelvicln=="Y"),
     data=hypox)
> fit
Call:
coxph(formula = Surv(dftime, dcens)~ifp + tumsize + (pelvicln
==''Y''), data = hypox)
```

```
                      coef  exp(coef)  se(coef)     z       p
ifp                 0.0617       1.06    0.0196  3.14  0.0017
tumsize             0.2301       1.26    0.1041  2.21  0.0270
pelvicln == "Y"TRUE 0.7436       2.10    0.4554  1.63  0.1000
```

```
Likelihood ratio test=19.9 on 3 df, p=0.000182 n= 109
```

As for the local relapse analysis, the p-values for the distant relapse are also significant (0.0013 for the unadjusted model and 0.0017 for the adjusted model). These results suggest that high IFP is an

Table 6.3 Association of IFP (adjusted) with local relapse and distant relapse.

	Competing risks regression		Cox proportional hazards	
	Coefficient	p-value	Coefficient	p-value
Local	0.033	0.058	0.043	0.032
Distant	0.040	0.035	0.062	0.0017

indication of more aggressive tumours. Table 6.3 gives a summary of the adjusted effect of IFP for local and distant relapse based on the two types of modelling: hazards of the subdistribution using the `crr` function and cause-specific hazards using `coxph`. Note that, for both endpoints, the coefficients increase when the cause-specific hazard is modelled. Thus, when the other events are ignored, the effects are larger for both the local and the distant relapse because the occurrence of one type of event obstructs the observation of the other type of event. This fact affects the modelling of the hazards of the subdistribution but not the modelling of the cause-specific hazard. The latter tests the 'pure' effect: the effect with respect to one endpoint as if the other one did not exist. Based on these results new hypotheses can be generated to address the questions put forward earlier in this section.

6.4   CHECKING THE MODEL ASSUMPTIONS

The main assumption when modelling data is the proportionality of hazards. When the Fine and Gray method is used, it is necessary that the hazards of the CIF are proportional, whereas in the Cox proportional hazard model, it is the cause-specific hazards that need to be proportional. If the covariate is continuous, the model also assumes that the relationship between the logarithm of the hazard and the covariate is linear.

6.4.1   Proportionality of the cause-specific hazards

A visual inspection of the plot of $\log(-\log(S))$ vs. $\log(\text{time})$ (Lawless, 1982) can give a hint as to whether the cause-specific hazards can be assumed to be proportional. In this case S is the Kaplan–Meier estimate when the only event considered is the event of interest; both the observations without an event as well as the competing risks are censored. Such a plot can be drawn for each of the levels of a covariate. If the two curves are parallel then the assumption is satisfied. In a more general setting, if the covariate is continuous, a Schoenfeld residuals plot against time indicates whether there is a departure from this assumption. More details on this topic can be found in Therneau and Grambsch (2000).

Take, for example, the covariates `age` and `stage` from the `follic` dataset. The event of interest is failure due to disease recurrence. Since the cause-specific hazard is being modelled, the competing risks are ignored. Figure 6.3 shows the two curves for the two levels in the variable `stage`. The curve for stage II is shifted upwards. A careful examination of the two curves shows that the difference on the y-axis is larger at small time values than at large time values. To make this more apparent vertical line segments are drawn at 1, 2 and 10 years. The code in R for obtaining this graph is:

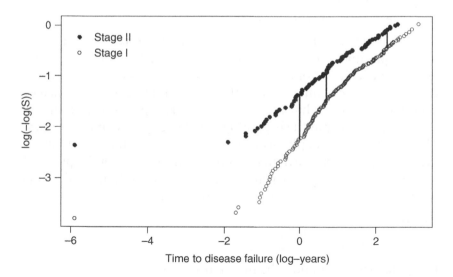

Figure 6.3 Proportionality of the cause-specific hazard for `stage` in the `follic` dataset: log–log graph.

```
> fit=survfit(Surv(follic$dftime,evcens)~stage)
> sumfit=summary(fit)
> lls0=log(-log(sumfit$surv[sumfit$strata=='stage=0']))
> t0=sumfit$time[sumfit$strata=='stage=0']
> plot(log(t0),lls0,xlab='Time to disease failure (log)',
        ylab='log(-log(S))')
> lls1=log(-log(sumfit$surv[sumfit$strata=='stage=1']))
> t1=sumfit$time[sumfit$strata=='stage=1']
> points(log(t1),lls1,pch=3)
```

The Schoenfeld residuals plot is much more convincing. It can be obtained using the function `cox.zph` in R. This function can be applied for different transformation of the x-axis. In the Figure 6.4a the identity transformation was chosen for which the x-axis is scaled based on the actual time. For the default transformation (km) x-axis is scaled using the $(1 - KM)$ estimate for the null model (Figure 6.4b). The km transformation is recommended because it is less sensitive to outliers and the points are evenly spread, but the x-axis is more difficult to interpret. Other possible transformations are `rank` (which is close to km) and `log`.

Figure 6.4A was obtained using the following commands:

```
> fit=coxph(Surv(follic$dftime,evcens)~stage)
> schfit=cox.zph(fit,transform='identity')
> plot(schfit[1])
> abline(h=fit$coef[1],lty=2)
```

By replacing the transformation with `transform='km'`, or leaving this parameter out, Figure 6.4b is created. The solid line is the estimated coefficient of `stage` over time, the dotted lines represent its 95% confidence interval, and the horizontal line is the coefficient if proportionality of hazards is assumed. The plot shows that the coefficient is larger at the beginning and decreases as time increases. The function `cox.zph` also gives a *p*-value which, if small, is evidence against proportional hazards. Both the look of the plot and the test of significance depend on the transformation used. Thus with `identity` transformation the results are:

```
> schfit
           rho   chisq       p
  stage  -0.192   10.0  0.00153
```

Using km transformation the function produces:

```
> schfit=cox.zph(fit)
> schfit
```

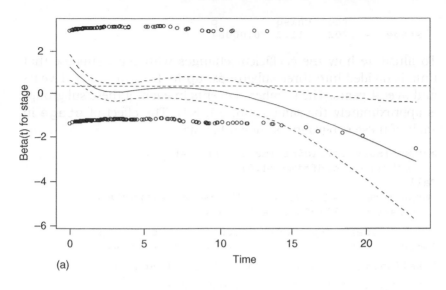

(a)

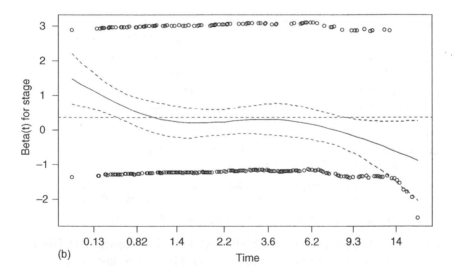

(b)

Figure 6.4 Proportionality of the cause-specific hazard for `stage` in the `follic` dataset: Schoenfeld residuals (a) using the identity transformation; (b) using the default transformation (km).

```
              rho   chisq        p
stage      -0.202   11.2   0.00084
```

To illustrate how the coefficient changes with time, suppose that time is divided into three subgroups: up to 1.5 years, 1.5–4 years and over 4 years. The number of events in each of these subgroups is approximately the same (106, 83, 83). The effect of stage in each of these subgroups is shown below:

```
> coxph(Surv(follic$dftime,evcens)~stage,
    sub=(follic$dftime<=1.5))
Call:
coxph(formula = Surv(follic$dftime, evcens)~stage,
    subset = (follic$dftime <= 1.5))

          coef   exp(coef)   se(coef)     z      p
stage    0.476        1.61      0.197   2.42  0.016

Likelihood ratio test=5.74 on 1 df, p=0.0166 n= 116
> coxph(Surv(follic$dftime,evcens)~stage,
        sub=(follic$dftime>1.5 & follic$dftime<=4))
Call:
coxph(formula = Surv(follic$dftime, evcens)~stage,
    subset = (follic$dftime > 1.5 & follic$dftime <= 4))

          coef   exp(coef)   se(coef)     z      p
stage    0.361        1.44      0.234   1.54   0.12

Likelihood ratio test=2.28 on 1 df, p=0.131 n= 107
> coxph(Surv(follic$dftime,evcens)~stage,
        sub=(follic$dftime>4))
Call:
coxph(formula = Surv(follic$dftime, evcens)~stage,
    subset = (follic$dftime > 4))

           coef   exp(coef)   se(coef)       z      p
stage   -0.0457       0.955      0.240  -0.190   0.85

Likelihood ratio test=0.04 on 1 df, p=0.849 n= 318
```

In the first subgroup the coefficient is 0.476, decreasing to 0.361 in the second subgroup and further to −0.046 in the last subgroup.

Age in the follic dataset is an example where the assumption of proportionality of hazards is satisfied. The result from cox.zph is:

```
               rho   chisq      p
follic$age  0.0286   0.205   0.65
```

The Schoenfeld residuals plot obtained using the km transformation is shown in Figure 6.5. The solid line, which represents the effect

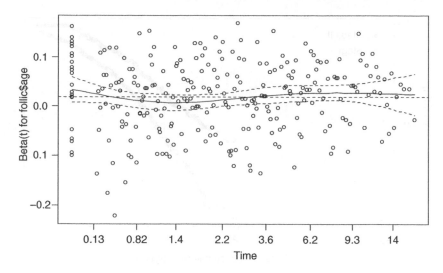

Figure 6.5 Proportionality of the cause-specific hazard for `age` in the `follic` dataset: Schoenfeld residuals.

of age over time, is fairly horizontal, suggesting proportionality of hazards.

6.4.2   Proportionality of the hazards of the CIF

To investigate the proportionality assumtion for the competing risks regression $\log\left(-\log\left(1-F\right)\right)$ can be plotted against $\log\left(\text{time}\right)$, where F is the CIF for the event of interest. Figure 6.6 illustrates such a plot for `stage` in the `follic` dataset for the failure due to disease. The R code is:

```
> fit=cuminc(follic$dftime,cens,stage)
> a=timepoints(fit,times=follic$dftime)
> cif=t(a$est[1:2,])
> llcif=log(-log(1-cif))
>
matplot(log(unique(sort(follic$dftime))),llcif,pch=c(1,3),
    col=1,
    xlab='Time to disease failure', ylab='log(-log(1-CIF))')
```

Note that the curves are slightly further apart at small time values. As shown in Section 6.2.3, a time-dependent covariate

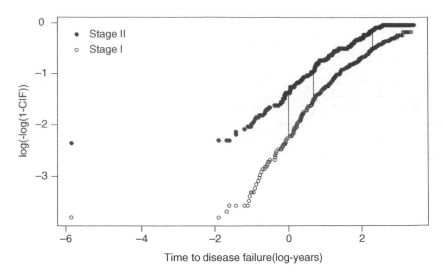

Figure 6.6 Proportionality of the hazard of the CIF for `stage` in the `follic` dataset: log–log graph.

can be included in the model, which tests whether the hazard ratio for stage changes with time. Figure 6.6 and the analysis in Section 6.2.3 agree, suggesting that the effect of the variable stage decreases with time.

6.4.3   Linearity assumption

In modelling the cause-specific hazard as well as the hazard of the CIF it is assumed that the logarithm of hazard changes linearly with the covariate. The assumption of linearity can be checked by categorizing the covariate and examining the coefficients for each category. If the coefficients increase linearly then the assumption is satisfied. Note that the number of categories is dictated by the size of the dataset and more precisely by the number of events present in the dataset.

In the `follic` dataset there are 541 observations with more than 250 events of interest (272 disease failures). Here the variable `age` is categorized into five groups, each with about 100 observations: up to 43, 43–55, 55–62, 62–69 and over 69. Let us create the four dummy variables needed:

```
> age4355=(follic$age>43 & follic$age<=55)+0
> age5562=(follic$age>55 & follic$age<=62)+0
> age6269=(follic$age>62 &follic$age<=69)+0
> age6986=(follic$age>69)+0
```

The model gives us the following results:

```
>crr(follic$dftime,cens,cbind(age4355,age5562,
  age6269,age6986))
convergence: TRUE
coefficients:
[1] 0.4518 0.5568 0.4685 0.6883
standard errors:
[1] 0.2061 0.2036 0.2165 0.2103
two-sided p-values:
[1] 0.0280 0.0062 0.0300 0.0011
```

Each of the coefficients represents the difference in the log-hazard of the CIF between the specific group and the baseline group (age up to 43). Using 0 for the baseline group these coefficients are depicted in Figure 6.7. It is clear that the three groups in the middle do not have a specific pattern. The oldest age group has higher hazard and the youngest has lower hazard. Fitting age and logarithm of age, we obtain:

```
> crr(follic$dftime,cens,follic$age)
convergence: TRUE
coefficients:
[1] 0.01339
standard errors:
[1] 0.004455
two-sided p-values:
[1] 0.0026
> crr(follic$dftime,cens,log(follic$age))
convergence: TRUE
coefficients:
[1] 0.7519
standard errors:
[1] 0.2373
two-sided p-values:
[1] 0.0015
```

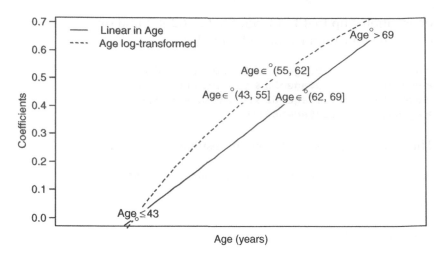

Figure 6.7 The linearity of age with the log of the hazard of the CIF.

The solid line in Figure 6.7 represents the linear fit of the covariate age. The dotted line is obtained using log-transformed age. The latter provides a slightly better fit. Since these results are data-driven and do not provide a strong evidence for the logarithmic model, it is preferable to choose the simple form (linear) for the time being.

The same method can be applied when the cause-specific hazard is modelled:

```
> coxph(Surv(follic$dftime,evcens)~age4355+age5562+age6269
  +age6986)
Call:
coxph(formula = Surv(follic$dftime, evcens)~age4355 + age5562
+ age6269 + age6986)
```

	coef	exp(coef)	se(coef)	z	p
age4355	0.491	1.63	0.207	2.37	1.8e-02
age5562	0.619	1.86	0.207	2.99	2.8e-03
age6269	0.612	1.84	0.216	2.84	4.5e-03
age6986	0.896	2.45	0.209	4.29	1.8e-05

```
Likelihood ratio test=20.5 on 4 df, p=0.000402 n= 541
```

The graph of these coefficients suggests that the log of the cause-specific hazard is approximately linear with age. When the cause-specific hazard is modelled, the martingale residuals (Therneau and Grambsch, 2000) can also be examined to determine the functional

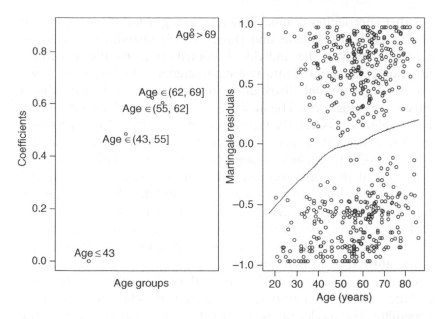

Figure 6.8 The linearity of `age` with the log of cause-specific hazard.

form of the covariate. This plot is created using the following commands:

```
> fit=coxph(Surv(follic$dftime,evcens)~1)
> plot(follic$age,resid(fit))
> lines(lowess(follic$age,resid(fit),iter=0))
```

As expected, the two plots (Figure 6.8) suggest that age is linear with log of the cause-specific hazard.

6.5 CLOSING REMARKS

This chapter has discussed the modelling of competing risk data. Two main approaches were introduced: modelling cause-specific hazard and modelling the hazard of the CIF. It has also discussed some ways to check the assumptions of the models. Although modelling small datasets is not recommended, several hypothetical examples with few observations were included for the purpose of illustrating the calculations. Real-life examples were also analysed.

Other approaches to modelling competing risk data are discussed in the literature. Larson and Dinse (1985) introduced a mixture model in which the individual contribution to the likelihood function is partitioned into two components: a logistic term based on the multinomial distribution of the types of failure and a survival-specific term. The model built in this way does not assume independence between the types of events. Tai *et al.* (2001) proposed modelling the CIF directly. This method was later extended (Tai *et al.*, 2002) to include observations with two types of events occurring at the same point in time. An extension of the Fine and Gray method from Section 6.2 was formulated by Fine (1999). In this approach, a logit transformation of the CIF is modelled. Although this model does not perform well when the hazard of the CIF is proportional, its benefit is the possibility of using it with many other transformations.

For the modelling of the hazard of the subdistribution the work of Fine and Gray (1999) was presented in detail because of its versatility. The model can be regarded as a natural extension of the Cox proportional hazards model, where the hazard is replaced by the hazard of the subdistribution. Hence, the interpretation of the coefficients is not dissimilar to that of the Cox model coefficients. The availability of software that can perform this type of analysis and the possibility of incorporating time-dependent covariates constitute a definite advantage.

Calculating the power in the presence of competing risks

7.1 INTRODUCTION

In the process of designing a study an important step is to calculate the sample size necessary to obtain a specific power at a specific significance level for the test used in the analysis. In other words, we wish to calculate a sample size which would minimize the two types of error: type I (α), which is the probability of obtaining a significant difference when in fact there is none; and type II (β), which is the probability of not detecting a true difference. The power of a study is defined as $1 - \beta$. To calculate the power one uses the minimum effect size that the researcher would not want to miss. For time-to-event analyses the effect size is expressed as the ratio of the hazards of the two arms, which is assumed to be constant over time.

In the presence of competing risks there are two types of hazard ratios that can be tested: the ratio of the cause-specific hazards and the ratio of the hazards of the subdistribution (Chapters 5 and 6). The calculation of sample size mirrors these two approaches of analysing the data in the presence of competing risks.

Competing Risks: A Practical Perspective   M. Pintilie
© 2006 John Wiley & Sons, Ltd

The sample size calculations are first reviewed for the case of no competing risks, and then presented for each of the two approaches used in the analysis of data in the presence of competing risks. It is assumed that the times to the two types of event follow an exponential distribution, and that the two types of events are independent. Some formulae are also given for the situation where the exponential distribution is not a valid assumption.

Denote by F the cumulative incidence function and by KM the Kaplan–Meier estimate, such that when there are no competing risks $F = 1 - KM$. All the calculations are performed for a study in which the population is divided evenly between the two arms. The subscript 0 is used for information referring to the standard arm and 1 for the experimental arm. Label the event of interest using the subscript ev and the competing risk using cr.

7.2 SAMPLE SIZE CALCULATION WHEN COMPETING RISKS ARE NOT PRESENT

Suppose that it is desired to calculate the necessary number of patients to detect a hazard ratio, θ, at the level of significance α with a power $1 - \beta$. The necessary number of events is given by:

$$n_{ev} = \left(\frac{z_{1-\alpha/2} + z_{1-\beta}}{\text{std}(x) \log(\theta)} \right)^2, \tag{7.1}$$

where z_α is the α quantile of the normal distribution and $\text{std}(x)$ is the standard deviation of the covariate x. If a randomized study is planned to compare two treatments, with the proportion of subjects in the standard treatment arm being π, then $\text{std}(x) = \sqrt{\pi(1 - \pi)}$. Usually, in practice, $\pi = 1/2$ then $\text{std}(x) = 1/2$ and

$$n_{ev} = \left(\frac{2(z_{1-\alpha/2} + z_{1-\beta})}{\log(\theta)} \right)^2.$$

The probability of an event occuring during the study period can be calculated, as shown in Collett (2003), by

$$P_{ev} = 1 - \frac{1}{a} \int_{f}^{a+f} S(u)du, \qquad (7.2)$$

where S is the survivor function, a is the duration of accrual and f is the follow-up time added at the end of accrual. If the time-to-event in the experimental arm follows an exponential distribution with parameter λ_1 then the formula becomes

$$P_{ev1} = 1 - \frac{e^{-\lambda_1 f} - e^{-\lambda_1 (a+f)}}{\lambda_1 a}. \qquad (7.3)$$

The probability of an event during the study period for the standard arm, P_{ev0}, can be calculated similarly.

If the exponential distribution cannot be assumed then equation (7.2) can be approximated using Simpson's rule (Collett, 2003). In this case the probability of an event occuring during the study period in the experimental group is

$$P_{ev1} = 1 - \frac{1}{6} \{ S_1(f) + 4S_1(0.5a+f) + S_1(a+f) \}. \qquad (7.4)$$

The probability of an event for the whole study is

$$P_{ev} = \pi P_{ev1} + (1 - \pi)P_{ev0} = \frac{P_{ev1} + P_{ev0}}{2}$$

and the total number of patients needed is $N = n_{ev}/P_{ev}$.

In practice, since the sample size is closely linked with the accrual time, it is easier to calculate the power for a specific sample size rather than the sample size to meet the specific power. Therefore the power calculation consists of two steps: calculation of the probability of observing an event during the study (equation (7.3) or (7.4)) and ultimately the number of events needed, n_{ev}; and then calculation of $z_{1-\beta}$ and therefore the power.

The use of median survival estimates as a measure for effect size is not recommended. In populations where the number of censored observations is not small, the median survival either does not exist or may be very unstable.

7.3 CALCULATING POWER IN THE PRESENCE OF COMPETING RISKS

7.3.1 General formulae

The presence of competing risks does not allow the observation of all possible events. Therefore, formulae (7.3) and (7.4) are different in this case. The probability of observing the event of interest during the study is given by:

$$P_{\mathrm{ev}} = 1 - \frac{1}{a} \int_f^{a+f} \{1 - F_{\mathrm{ev}}(u)\}\, du \qquad (7.5)$$

where F_{ev} is the CIF for the event of interest, a is accrual time and f is the follow-up time. Solving the integral for the experimental group gives:

$$P_{\mathrm{ev1}} = \frac{\lambda_{\mathrm{ev1}}}{\lambda_{\mathrm{ev1}} + \lambda_{\mathrm{cr1}}} \left(1 - \frac{e^{-(\lambda_{\mathrm{ev1}} + \lambda_{\mathrm{cr1}})f} - e^{-(\lambda_{\mathrm{ev1}} + \lambda_{\mathrm{cr1}})(a+f)}}{(\lambda_{\mathrm{ev1}} + \lambda_{\mathrm{cr1}})a} \right). \qquad (7.6)$$

A similar expression results for the standard group. Then the overall probability of a patient experiencing an event during the entire study is $P_{\mathrm{ev}} = \pi P_{\mathrm{ev1}} + (1 - \pi)P_{\mathrm{ev0}}$ and the expected number of events for the sample size N is $n_{\mathrm{ev}} = N \times P_{\mathrm{ev}}$.

For the second part of this calculation formula (7.1) gives

$$z_{1-\beta} = \sqrt{n_{\mathrm{ev}}\pi(1-\pi)}\ \log(\theta) - z_{1-\alpha/2}. \qquad (7.7)$$

The above formula is the same regardless whether the aim is to compare the cause-specific hazards or the hazards of the CIF. In the former case θ represents the ratio of the cause-specific hazards, while in the latter case it represents the ratio of the hazards of the CIFs. To avoid confusion, in this chapter, the ratio of the cause-specific hazards for the event of interest will henceforth be denoted by θ, while the ratio of the hazards of the CIFs for the event of interest will be denoted by θ_F.

These calculations require knowledge of the total number of patients (N) that can be accrued in the accrual time (a), the effect size (θ or θ_F), the hazards for the event of interest and for competing risks for both groups (λ_{ev0}, λ_{cr0}, λ_{ev1} and λ_{cr1}) and the follow-up time (f). In practical situations the accrual time, the follow-up time and the total number of patients are known. The effect size may be known either as a hazard ratio or as the estimates of the probability of an event in the two groups at a certain point in time, or even as Kaplan–Meier estimates at a point in time in the two groups. The next section is concerned with the effect size (when unknown) and the hazards for the event of interest and competing risks in the two groups in the two main scenarios: when cause-specific hazards are compared and when hazards of the subdistributions are compared.

7.3.2   Comparing cause-specific hazards

Comparison of cause-specific hazards depends on what is known at time t.

θ, KM_{ev0} and KM_{cr0} known

The hazard rates for the event of interest and for the competing risks can easily be obtained from the Kaplan–Meier estimates:

$$\lambda_{ev0} = \frac{\log(KM_{ev0})}{t} \tag{7.8a}$$

and, similarly,

$$\lambda_{cr0} = \frac{\log(KM_{cr0})}{t}. \tag{7.8b}$$

Since $\theta = \lambda_{ev0}/\lambda_{ev1}$, it follows that $\lambda_{ev1} = \lambda_{ev0}/\theta$. It is assumed that the competing risks are similar in the two groups, therefore $\lambda_{cr1} = \lambda_{cr0}$.

$KM_{ev0}, KM_{cr0}, KM_{ev1}$ and KM_{cr1} known

Using (7.8), the hazards λ_{ev0}, λ_{cr0}, λ_{ev1} and λ_{cr1} can easily be obtained. The effect size is then $\theta = \lambda_{ev0}/\lambda_{ev1}$.

θ, F_{ev0} and F_{cr0} known

The hazard rates for the standard arm can be found by solving the following system of equations (Pintilie, 2002):

$$F_{ev0} = \frac{\lambda_{ev0}}{\lambda_{ev0} + \lambda_{cr0}}(1 - e^{-(\lambda_{ev0} + \lambda_{cr0})t}),$$

$$F_{cr0} = \frac{\lambda_{cr0}}{\lambda_{ev0} + \lambda_{cr0}}(1 - e^{-(\lambda_{ev0} + \lambda_{cr0})t}). \tag{7.9}$$

This has solution

$$\lambda_{ev0} = F_{ev0}(t) \times \frac{-\ln(1 - F_{ev0}(t) - F_{cr0}(t))}{t(F_{ev0}(t) + F_{cr0}(t))},$$

$$\lambda_{cr0} = F_{cr0}(t) \times \frac{-\ln(1 - F_{ev0}(t) - F_{cr0}(t))}{t(F_{ev0}(t) + F_{cr0}(t))}. \tag{7.10}$$

As before, $\lambda_{ev1} = \lambda_{ev0}/\theta$ and $\lambda_{cr1} = \lambda_{cr0}$.

$F_{ev0}, F_{cr0}, F_{ev1}$ and F_{cr1} known

The hazard rates are obtained by solving (7.9) for the standard arm and then for the experimental arm. As usual, $\theta = \lambda_{ev0}/\lambda_{ev1}$.

7.3.3   Comparing hazards of the subdistributions

Comparison of hazards of the subdistributions again depends on what is known at time t.

θ_F, KM_{ev0} and KM_{cr0} known

The hazard rates λ_{ev0} and λ_{cr0} can be calculated using (7.8), based on which F_{ev0} and F_{cr0} can be obtained from (7.9). Since

$$\theta_F = \frac{\log(1 - F_{ev0})}{\log(1 - F_{ev1})}, \tag{7.11}$$

it follows that $F_{ev1} = 1 - (1 - F_{ev0})^{1/\theta_F}$. It is also assumed that the competing risks do not change, that is, $\lambda_{cr1} = \lambda_{cr0}$. Note that this does not imply that $F_{cr1} = F_{cr0}$. This would be an unreasonable assumption since F_{cr1} depends on both λ_{ev1} (which is different from λ_{ev0}) and λ_{cr1}. The parameter λ_{ev1} can be obtained by solving the equation

$$F_{ev1} = \frac{\lambda_{ev1}}{\lambda_{ev1} + \lambda_{cr1}}(1 - e^{-(\lambda_{ev1} + \lambda_{cr1})t}). \qquad (7.12)$$

This equation is transcendental and can be solved using numerical methods.

KM_{ev0}, KM_{cr0}, KM_{ev1} and KM_{cr1} known

The hazard rates $\lambda_{ev0}, \lambda_{cr0}, \lambda_{ev1}$ and λ_{cr1} can be calculated using (7.8), and then F_{ev0} and F_{ev1} can be obtained. The hazard ratio θ_F is given by (7.11).

θ_F, F_{ev0} and F_{cr0} known

Since θ_F is known, $F_{ev1} = 1 - (1 - F_{ev0})^{1/\theta_F}$ can be found as before. The parameters λ_{ev0} and λ_{cr0} can be calculated using (7.10), but λ_{ev1} needs to be calculated by solving (7.12) using numerical methods.

F_{ev0}, F_{cr0}, F_{ev1} and F_{cr1} known

The system of equations (7.9) and (7.10) can be applied for each group to give $\lambda_{ev0}, \lambda_{cr0}, \lambda_{ev1}$ and λ_{cr1}. The hazard ratio θ_F is given by (7.11).

7.3.4 Probability of event when the exponential distribution is not a valid assumption

When the exponential distribution is not a valid assumption, the probability of a patient experiencing an event during the study (formula (7.5)) can be approximated using Simpson's rule by

$$P_{ev} = \frac{1}{6}\{F_{ev}(f) + 4F_{ev}(f + 0.5a) + F_{ev}(a + f)\}, \qquad (7.13)$$

where F_{ev} is the CIF for the event of interest. Note that the use of this formula is limited by the need for a good estimate for the CIF at $a + f$. To appreciate how difficult this is, an example is provided. Suppose that a power calculation is needed for a study, which is planned to accrue patients over a 5-year period. Two extra years of follow-up will be added after finishing accrual. This is a common requirement. However, to apply Simpson's rule we need to have a good estimate of the CIF at 7 years, which means that this information needs to be drawn from a study for which the median follow-up is at least 5 or 6 years, so that the 7-year estimate is reasonably stable.

7.4 EXAMPLES

7.4.1 Introduction

The R function `power`, which can be found in Appendix B, helps calculate the power. It is assumed that the time to each type of event in each group follows an exponential distribution and that the time to event and time to competing risk are independent. If the Kaplan–Meier or CIF estimates are available only for the standard arm (subscript 0) then the hazard rate for the competing risk for the experimental arm is considered the same as for the standard arm. Otherwise it is calculated from the estimates for the experimental arm (subscript 1).

7.4.2 Comparing the cause-specific hazard

The hypoxia trial suggested that patients with hypoxic tumors (HP5 > 50) were more likely to experience a failure. The researchers wish to try a new drug which has a selective toxicity for hypoxic cells, hoping in this way to improve the rate for local failure. Since the goal of the study is to test the effect of the drug at the cell level, the analysis will be based on the cause-specific hazard ratio. Let us plan a two-arm randomized study: standard treatment (radiation and cysplatin) vs. the experimental treatment (radiation, cysplatin and the new drug). It is desirable to detect a twofold decrease in the cause-specific hazard ratio (HR = 2) due to the new drug at the level of significance $\alpha = 0.05$ (two-sided). It is assumed that about 50 patients per year can be accrued over a period of 3 years, with 2 extra years of follow-up. The patients will be divided equally between the two arms. Suppose that the Kaplan–Meier estimate for the event of interest at 3 years is 0.5 and the Kaplan–Meier estimate for the competing risks at 3 years is 0.4, then

```
> power(N=150, a=3, f=2, pi=0.5,theta=2, t0=3, KMev0=0.5, KMcr0=0.4)
[1] 0.6162274
```

If instead of the Kaplan–Meier estimates the CIF estimates are available, the same function can be applied:

```
> power(N=150, a=3, f=2, pi=0.5, theta=2, t0=3,
        CIFev0=0.345, CIFcr0=0.455)
[1] 0.6168332
```

Suppose that the treatment is expected to have an impact on competing risks such that the Kaplan–Meier estimate at 3 years in the experimental arm for the competing risk is 0.3 and the CIF at 3 years in the experimental arm is 0.61. Using the Kaplan–Meier estimate, the power is

```
> power(N=150, a=3, f=2, pi=0.5, t0=3,
        KMev0=0.5, KMcr0=0.4, KMev1=0.706, KMcr1=0.3)
[1] 0.5924636
```

while using the CIF estimates gives

```
> power(N=150, a=3, f=2, pi=0.5, t0=3,
        CIFev0=0.345, CIFcr0=0.455, CIFev1=0.177, CIFcr1=0.61)
[1] 0.5958667
```

The differences between the power calculated using the KM estimates and the power calculated using the CIF (0.616 227 4 and 0.616 833 2, or 0.592 463 6 and 0.595 866 7) are due to the approximation of the CIF and KM estimates imputed in the function `power`.

Note that the power when the competing risks are ignored is larger:

```
> power(N=150, a=3, f=2, pi=0.5, t0=3,
        KMev0=0.5, KMcr0=1, KMev1=0.706, KMcr1=1)
[1] 0.7969974
```

By applying the function power repeatedly one can estimate the number of patients needed to detect a certain effect size with a prespecified power. Suppose that the effect size to be detected is 2 and that it is desirable to have at least 80% power. The function applied for $N = 200$ calculates a power of 76%. With 250 patients the power becomes 85%. Since it is assumed that the rate of accrual is 50 per year the accrual of 250 takes 5 years.

```
> power(N=200, a=4, f=2, pi=0.5, theta=2, t0=3, KMev0=0.5, KMcr0=0.4)
[1] 0.7568012
> power(N=250, a=5, f=2, pi=0.5, theta=2, t0=3, KMev0=0.5, KMcr0=0.4)
[1] 0.8538274
```

With only 150 patients a larger effect size of 2.5 can be detected with 82% power:

```
> power(N=150, a=3, f=2, pi=0.5, theta=2.5, t0=3, KMev0=0.5, KMcr0=0.4)
[1] 0.8224128
```

7.4.3   Comparing the hazard of the subdistribution

Hodgkin's disease is one of the success stories of cancer treatment. The probability of cause-specific death at 5 and 10 years is about 10% and 15%, respectively. Hodgkin's disease is a disease specific to a younger population (median age is 30). Therefore, this population is ideal for studying the long-term side effects of cancer treatment. Suppose that there exists a cohort of 1000 Hodgkin's disease patients diagnosed and treated between 1981 and 1990. The standard treatment was either radiation or chemotherapy. The hypothesis is that administering radiation to the heart may increase the risk of heart failure. For the sake of this calculation it is assumed that roughly the same number and the same type of patients are treated with radiation to the chest (containing a portion of the heart) and with chemotherapy. The intention is to test whether the risk of heart failure increases due to radiation given to the heart. For this purpose precise details of the treatment as well as a very good follow-up for the detection of heart failures are needed. Therefore, although the cohort consists of 1000 records which fit the inclusion criteria, it is desirable to use no more than the necessary number of records. It is estimated that the risk of heart failure in this population at 10 years is 5%. It would be useful to be able to detect an increase of 5% between those treated with chest radiation (R) and those treated with chemotherapy (C). Assume that the incidence of competing risks at 10 years is 15% in the R group and 13% in the C group. The accrual time is 10 years and the follow-up time is 12 years. If 600 records are randomly selected from the cohort of 1000 then the power exceeds 80% at $\alpha = 0.05$ (two-sided):

```
> power(N=600,a=10,f=12,pi=0.5,t0=10,
        CIFev0=0.1,CIFcr0=0.13,CIFev1=0.05,CIFcr1=0.15)
[1] 0.845907
```

If the competing risks are ignored the power is slightly larger:

```
> power(N=600,a=10,f=12,pi=0.5,t0=10,
        CIFev0=0.1,CIFcr0=0,CIFev1=0.05,CIFcr1=0)
[1] 0.8724947
```

7.5 CLOSING REMARKS

This chapter has described methods for calculating the sample size when competing risks are present. The focus has been on the two situations specific to competing risks: comparing the cause-specific hazard and comparing the hazard of the subdistribution. Among the assumptions made were: uniform accrual, exponential distribution, independence between the time to event and the time to competing risks, and proportionality of hazards. It is not hard to recognize that the hazards of the subdistributions under the exponential distribution are not always proportional. Although the power calculation may seem of limited use in this case, it is known that for certain values of $\lambda_{ev0}, \lambda_{cr0}, \lambda_{ev1}$ and λ_{cr1} the ratio of the hazard of the subdistribution does not vary greatly with time. For example, for time less than $10, \lambda_{ev0} = 0.2, \lambda_{cr0} = 0.75, \lambda_{ev1} = 0.4$ and $\lambda_{cr1} = 0.58$ or $\lambda_{ev0} = 0.2, \lambda_{cr0} = 0.05, \lambda_{ev1} = 0.4$ and $\lambda_{cr1} = 0.015$ the ratio of hazards varies between 2 and 2.4. Furthermore, the ratios of the cumulative hazards of the subdistributions are much more stable (between 2.12 and 2.13 for the first case and between 2.04 and 2.25 for the second case). It would be valuable to find a theoretical distribution which would explain medical data well and would exhibit the desirable effect of proportionality of hazards. Then the exponential distribution could be replaced by a more reasonable model. Yet another alternative would be to obtain good estimates of the CIF for several time points for the standard arm. The estimates for the experimental arm would then be easily obtained using the formula $F_{ev1} = 1 - (1 - F_{ev0})^{1/\theta_F}$ and a similar one for the competing risks. All these estimates would facilitate the calculation of the probability of event using Simpson's rule (7.13).

8

Other issues in competing risks

8.1 CONDITIONAL PROBABILITY FUNCTION

8.1.1 Introduction

Previous chapters have indicated that the cumulative incidence function for the event of interest does not offer a complete understanding of competing risks data. It has to be augmented with the information given by the CIF for the competing risk. The reason for this recommendation is the fact that the CIF for the event of interest may appear low only because the CIF for the competing risk is large. Calculating the conditional probability (CP) is one way to incorporate the two types of information: event of interest and competing risk. The CP calculated at a time point, t, is the probability of observing an event of interest by time t, conditional on the individual not experiencing a competing risk event by time t. In the `follic` dataset let us consider two types of event: failure due to disease (relapse or no response to treatment) and death while in remission. The event of interest is the disease failure. The CIF at 10 years gives the probability of disease failure by 10 years, while the CP at 10 years is the probability of disease failure knowing that the patient had survived for that period of time. In general the CP

Competing Risks: A Practical Perspective M. Pintilie
© 2006 John Wiley & Sons, Ltd

of event i occurring by time t, given that no other type of event has occurred by then, is defined as

$$CP_i(t) = P(T \leq t, C = i \,|\, \text{no other type of event by } t).$$

Without any loss of generality, it can be assumed that there are only two types of events: the event of interest (ev) and the competing risk (cr). Then the CP for the event of interest can be expressed as

$$CP(t) = \frac{P(T \leq t, C = ev)}{1 - P(T \leq t, C = cr)} = \frac{F_{ev}(t)}{1 - F_{cr}(t)},$$

where F_{ev} and F_{cr} are the CIFs corresponding to the event of interest and competing risk, respectively. Like the CIF, the CP is an increasing monotonic function ranging between 0 and 1. Note that $CP(t) \geq F_{ev}(t)$ for any t.

8.1.2 Nonparametric estimation of the CP function

An estimator for CP can easily be obtained by using the estimators for F_{ev} and F_{cr} provided in Chapter 4:

$$\widehat{CP}(t) = \frac{\hat{F}_{ev}(t)}{1 - \hat{F}_{cr}(t)}. \tag{8.1}$$

The calculation of CP is illustrated on the hypothetical example given in Table 4.2. The event of interest is the injurious fall, coded as 1, and the rest of the events are considered competing risks (here coded as 2). The last column in Table 8.1 gives the CP estimates. Note that the CP changes not only when an event of interest is observed but also when a competing risk occurs.

8.1.3 Variance of the CP function estimator

As in the case of the CIF estimator, the exact variance of the CP function estimator is difficult to obtain. The estimator for the variance given by Pepe and Mori (1993) is presented below.

Table 8.1 Calculating $\hat{CP}(t)$ for event of interest (coded as 1) and competing risk (coded as 2).

Time to event (months)	Type of Event*	$\hat{F}_{ev}(t)$	$\hat{F}_{cr}(t)$	$\hat{CP}(t)$
0	—	0.0000	0.0000	$0.0/(1-0.0000) = 0.0000$
24	2	0.0000	0.1000	$0.0/(1-0.1000) = 0.0000$
37	0	0.0000	0.1000	$0.0/(1-0.1000) = 0.0000$
49	1	0.1125	0.1000	$0.1125/(1-0.1000) = 0.1250$
61	2	0.1125	0.2125	$0.1125/(1-0.2125) = 0.1429$
65	2	0.1125	0.3250	$0.1125/(1-0.3250) = 0.1667$
80	1			
80	2	0.2250	0.4375	$0.2250/(1-0.4375) = 0.4000$
106	2	0.2250	0.5500	$0.2250/(1-0.5500) = 0.5000$
113	0	0.2250	0.5500	$0.2250/(1-0.5500) = 0.5000$
128	1	0.4500	0.5500	$0.4500/(1-0.5500) = 1.0000$

* $1 =$ Event of interest, $2 =$ Competing risk event, $0 =$ No event.

Let $t_1 < t_2 < \ldots < t_r$ be the unique ordered time points when either the event of interest or the competing risk was observed. Denote by n_j, d_j and d_{evj}, respectively, the number at risk, the number of all types of events and the number of events of interest at time t_j. Then, an estimator for the variance of the CP is:

$$\hat{V}\left(\hat{CP}(t_j)\right) = \frac{\hat{S}(t_{j-1})^2}{[1-\hat{F}_{cr}(t_j)]^4} \sum_{t_i \le t_j} \frac{d_{evi}[1-\hat{F}_{cr}(t_i)]^2 + [\hat{F}_{ev}(t_i)]^2(d_i - d_{evi})}{n_i(n_i-1)},$$

(8.2)

where F_{ev} and F_{cr} are the estimates for the CIF for the event of interest and for the competing risk respectively, and $\hat{S}$ is the Kaplan–Meier estimate for the probability of being free of any event. Pepe and Mori showed that $\hat{CP}$ is asymptotically normal with variance given by (8.2).

As shown in Sections 2.3.1 and 4.2.4, the $100(1 - \alpha)\%$ confidence interval for $\hat{CP}$ can be obtained in two ways. The simple approach is given by the formula

$$\hat{CP}(t) \pm z_{1-\alpha/2}\sqrt{\hat{V}(\hat{CP}(t))},$$

where z_α is the α quantile of the standard normal distribution. As was the case for the CIF and for the survivor function, this confidence interval may result in bounds outside the range $[0, 1]$. To avoid this nuisance, the $\log(-\log)$ transformation can be used (Section A.2) resulting in the confidence interval $\left[\widehat{CP}(t)\right]^{\exp[\pm A]}$, where

$$A = \frac{z_{1-\alpha/2}\sqrt{\hat{V}(\widehat{CP}(t))}}{\widehat{CP}(t)\log(\widehat{CP}(t))}.$$

8.1.4 Testing a covariate

The test formulated by Pepe and Mori (1993) for the comparison between two CIFs (Chapter 5) is more general and can also be applied to the comparison between the CP functions between two groups. The test is based on a weighted sum of the direct differences between CP functions for the two groups. The form of the score statistic is

$$s = \sqrt{\frac{N_1 N_2}{N_1 + N_2}} \int_0^\tau W(t)\{CP_1(t) - CP_2(t)\}\,dt,$$

where N_1 and N_2 are the total numbers of subjects, $W(t)$ is a weight function and τ is the maximum time observed in the two groups, For the discrete case the formula for the score is

$$s = \sqrt{\frac{N_1 N_2}{N_1 + N_2}} \sum_{\text{all } t_j} \left\{ W(t_j)\left[\widehat{CP}_1(t_j) - \widehat{CP}_2(t_j)\right](t_{j+1} - t_j)\right\},$$

where the weight is given by

$$W(t_j) = \frac{(N_1 + N_2)\,\hat{C}_1(t_{j-1})\,\hat{C}_2(t_{j-1})}{N_1\hat{C}_1(t_{j-1}) + N_2\hat{C}_2(t_{j-1})}.$$

As in Chapter 5, N_1 and N_2 are the number of observations in each of the two groups and $1 - \hat{C}(t)$ is the estimate of the censoring distribution using the Kaplan–Meier method. The calculation of the score s is shown for an example in Table 8.2.

The variance estimator for the score s is

$$\hat{\sigma}^2 = \frac{N_1 N_2 \left(\hat{\sigma}_1^2 + \hat{\sigma}_2^2 \right)}{N_1 + N_2},$$

where $\hat{\sigma}_1$ and $\hat{\sigma}_2$ are the estimates for the variances for each of the two groups. Each of these variances can be estimated using the

Table 8.2 Example for the calculation of the test for CP formulated by Pepe and Mori. $N_1 = 13, N_2 = 7$.

Time	Events*	Group	$\widehat{CP}_1(t)$	$\widehat{CP}_2(t)$	$W(t)$	$W(\widehat{CP}_1 - \widehat{CP}_2)$ $(t_{j+1} - t_j)$
1	2	2	0.0000	0.0000	1.0000	0.0000
2	2	1	0.0000	0.0000	0.9023	0.0000
3	0	1	0.0000	0.0000	0.8791	0.0000
4	1	2	0.0000	0.1667	0.8533	−0.1422
5	1	1	0.0909	0.1667	0.8533	−0.0646
6	0	1	0.0909	0.1667	0.8533	−0.0646
7	2	2	0.0909	0.2	0.8211	−0.0896
8	0	1	0.0909	0.2	0.7105	−0.0775
9	1	2	0.0909	0.4	0.6826	−0.211
10	0	1	0.0909	0.4	0.6826	−0.211
11	2	1	0.1045	0.4	0.6498	−0.192
12	1	1	0.2537	0.4	0.6108	−0.0893
13	1	1	0.4030	0.4	0.6108	0.0018
14	2	1	0.4737	0.4	0.6108	0.045
15	2	2	0.4737	0.5	0.5356	−0.0141
16	1	1	0.6491	0.5	0.4272	0.0637
17	1	2	0.6491	0.75	0.4272	−0.0431
18	1	1	0.8246	0.75	0.4272	0.0318
19	0	1	—	—	—	—
20	0	2	—	—	—	—
						Total $= -1.0567$
						$s = -2.2541$

* $1 =$ Event of interest, $2 =$ Competing risk event, $0 =$ No event.

formulae given below in which the subscript for the group (1 or 2) is omitted.

$$\hat{\sigma}^2 = \sum_{\text{all } t_j} \left[v\left(t_j\right) \right]^2 \frac{\left[1 - \hat{F}_{\text{cr}}\left(t_j\right)\right]^2 d_{\text{ev}j} + \left[\hat{F}_{\text{ev}}\left(t_j\right)\right]^2 \left(d_j - d_{\text{ev}j}\right)}{n_j \left(n_j - 1\right)},$$

where

$$v\left(t_j\right) = \sum_{t_k \geq t_j} \frac{W\left(t_k\right) \hat{S}\left(t_k\right)}{\left(1 - \hat{F}_{\text{ev}}\left(t_k\right)\right)^2} \left(t_{k+1} - t_k\right).$$

The extension of this test to k groups (Lunn, 1998) mentioned in Chapter 5 can also be applied for CP functions.

8.1.5   Using R

The bone marrow transplant data, bmt, introduced in Section 1.6.4, is used here as an example. Let us calculate the conditional probability of observing chronic graft vs. host disease (CGVHD) knowing that the patient was alive and did not experience a relapse. Figure 4.3 depicts the CIFs for each of these three types of events. Assume that CGVHD is the event of interest and that relapse and death represent the competing risks. Since each patient recorded as dead had experienced either CGVHD or relapse, death is not a competing risk. As in Chapter 4, first create the variable representing the time to first event

```
> bmt$dftime=apply(cbind(bmt$cgvhtime,bmt$reltime,bmt$survtime)
  ,1,min)
```

and the censoring variable

```
> cens=(bmt$dftime==bmt$cgvhtime & bmt$cgvh==1)+
  2*(bmt$dftime==bmt$reltime & bmt$rcens==1)+
  2*(bmt$dftime==bmt$survtime & bmt$stat==1)
```

Using the function CPvar from Appendix B, the conditional probabilities for the two treatment groups and their variances can be calculated. Since the number of events is quite large, the output is given here only up to 0.4 years:

```
> fit=CPvar(bmt$dftime,cens,bmt$tx)
> fit
[[1]]
```

	time	cif	fcr	cp	varCP	group
3	0.110	0.00	0.02	0.00000000	0.0000000000	BM
4	0.172	0.00	0.04	0.00000000	0.0000000000	BM
5	0.181	0.00	0.06	0.00000000	0.0000000000	BM
6	0.219	0.00	0.08	0.00000000	0.0000000000	BM
7	0.274	0.00	0.10	0.00000000	0.0000000000	BM
8	0.277	0.02	0.10	0.02222222	0.0005050505	BM
9	0.279	0.04	0.10	0.04444444	0.0009881647	BM
11	0.287	0.06	0.12	0.06818182	0.0015638099	BM
12	0.290	0.10	0.12	0.11363636	0.0024806065	BM
13	0.301	0.12	0.14	0.13953488	0.0030265588	BM
14	0.307	0.14	0.14	0.16279070	0.0032799579	BM
15	0.320	0.16	0.14	0.18604651	0.0036613440	BM
18	0.331	0.18	0.14	0.20930233	0.0040175009	BM
21	0.345	0.22	0.14	0.25581395	0.0049056525	BM
23	0.350	0.26	0.14	0.30232558	0.0054620497	BM
24	0.359	0.28	0.14	0.32558140	0.0053601119	BM
27	0.372	0.30	0.14	0.34883721	0.0055688751	BM
28	0.375	0.32	0.14	0.37209302	0.0057523003	BM
30	0.381	0.34	0.14	0.39534884	0.0059103929	BM

```
...
```

```
[[2]]
```

	time	cif	fcr	cp	varCP	group
2	0.063	0.00000000	0.02040816	0.00000000	0.000000000	PB
8	0.277	0.08163265	0.02040816	0.08333333	0.001773050	PB
10	0.282	0.10204082	0.02040816	0.10416667	0.001933976	PB
11	0.287	0.12244898	0.02040816	0.12500000	0.002291428	PB
15	0.320	0.14285714	0.02040816	0.14583333	0.002630703	PB
16	0.323	0.16326531	0.02040816	0.16666667	0.002951802	PB
17	0.329	0.20408163	0.02040816	0.20833333	0.003699881	PB
18	0.331	0.22448980	0.02040816	0.22916667	0.003784901	PB
19	0.339	0.24489796	0.02040816	0.25000000	0.004034401	PB
20	0.342	0.26530612	0.02040816	0.27083333	0.004265700	PB
22	0.348	0.28571429	0.02040816	0.29166667	0.004478802	PB
25	0.361	0.30612245	0.02040816	0.31250000	0.004673707	PB
26	0.367	0.36734694	0.02040816	0.37500000	0.005745599	PB
29	0.378	0.38775510	0.02040816	0.39583333	0.005197423	PB
30	0.381	0.40816327	0.02040816	0.41666667	0.005306232	PB
31	0.383	0.42857143	0.02040816	0.43750000	0.005396697	PB
32	0.392	0.44897959	0.02040816	0.45833333	0.005468824	PB

```
33  0.394 0.46938776 0.02040816 0.47916667 0.005522616 PB
34  0.397 0.48979592 0.02040816 0.50000000 0.005558081 PB
...
```

The plot is given in Figure 8.1 and can be obtained using the function `plot.cp`:

```
> plot.cp(fit, xlab='Time to CGVHD (years)',
  ylab='Probability of CGVHD conditioned on relapse and death')
```

Figures 5.3 and 5.4 suggest that for the `follic` dataset the observation of relapse in the older population is hindered by the occurrence of death. The conditional probabilities of relapse in the two groups (Figure 8.2) confirm this. Note that the two curves are well separated. By applying the Pepe–Mori test for conditional probability, using the function `compCP` from Appendix B, a *p*-value of 0.000 15 is found:

```
> a=(follic$age>65)+0
> compCP(follic$dftime,cens,a)
  chisquare          pvalue
   14.31814   0.0001543702
```

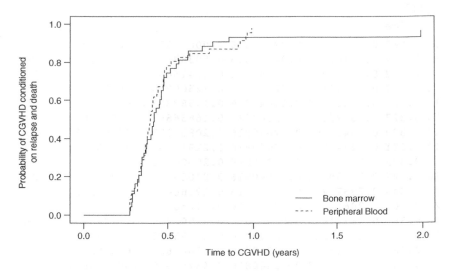

Figure 8.1 Conditional probability for the `bmt` dataset by treatment arm.

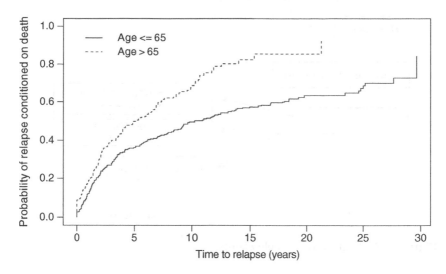

Figure 8.2 Conditional probability for the `follic` dataset by `age`.

Another measure of interest for clinicians is the probability of an individual experiencing the event of interest within a time frame assuming that the patient had not experienced any other types of events at the beginning of the period. For example, the probability of an individual in the `follic` dataset experiencing a relapse between 3 and 5 years since diagnosis can be estimated, given that at 3 years the patient was alive and well. Figure 8.3 shows the possible events. By 3 years a patient could have had a relapse (the set R_3) or died (the set D_3) or could have been alive and well (the rest of the diagram: R_{3-5}, D_{3-5}, A_5). The last set could be divided further. A patient alive and well at 3 years could have a relapse between 3 and 5 years (the set R_{3-5}) or die between 3 and 5 years (the set D_{3-5}) or could be alive and well at the end of the 5-year period (the set A_5). Thus the probability of experiencing a relapse between 3 and 5 years given that the patient was alive and well at 3 years can be calculated as follows:

$$P(R_{3-5}|A_3) = \frac{P(R_{3-5} \cap A_3)}{P(A_3)} = \frac{P(R_{3-5})}{P(A_3)}$$

$$= \frac{P(R_{3-5})}{1 - P(R_3) - P(D_3)} = \frac{F_{ev}(5) - F_{ev}(3)}{1 - F_{ev}(3) - F_{cr}(3)},$$

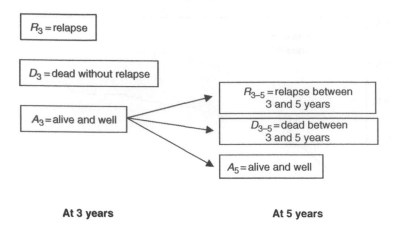

Figure 8.3 Diagram of possible events.

where F_{ev} is the CIF for relapse and F_{cr} is the CIF for death without relapse.

The CIF for relapse and for death without relapse at 3 and 5 years can be estimated using the function cuminc:

```
> fit=cuminc(follic$dftime,cens)
> sumfit=timepoints(fit,times=c(3,5))
> sumfit
$est
                3             5
1  1  0.29794800  0.37737381
1  2  0.03147720  0.05235004

$var
                3             5
1  1  3.880660e-04  4.390311e-04
1  2  5.658369e-05  9.304998e-05
```

The probability of relapse between 3 and 5 years given that the patient was alive and well at 3 years can be calculated using the estimates in sumfit$est:

```
> (sumfit$est[1,2]-sumfit$est[1,1])/(1-sumfit$est[1,1]-
sumfit$est[2,1])
[1] 0.1184444
```

For a patient in this dataset there is about a 12% chance of having a relapse between 3 and 5 years knowing that he/she was alive and well at 3 years. The variance of this estimate and its 95% confidence interval can be calculated by applying the bootstrap procedure `btvarCP2` (Appendix B). With 2000 bootstrap repetitions and the seed 2, the following result is obtained (which can be replicated if the same seed is used): replicate the result

```
> btvarCP2(follic$dftime,cens,3,5,2000,s0=2,alpha=0.05)
      CPw          varCPw        L95.CI      U95.CI
  0.1184444    0.0002880296    0.08773179   0.1540965
```

The 95% confidence interval is (9%,15%). Only the variance and the 95% confidence interval are estimated using the bootstrap. If one is interested only in the estimation of the probability, one could apply the bootstrap procedure for just one repetition:

```
> btvarCP2(follic$dftime,cens,3,5,1,s0=2,alpha=0.05)
      CPw    varCPw    L95.CI    U95.CI
  0.1184444     NA        NA        NA
```

8.1.6 Using SAS

The SAS macro `cuminc` calculates the CIFs for the event of interest and the competing risk as well as the conditional probability, together with their variances. The macro also plots the CIFs and CP curves. The macro `compcp` tests the difference between two CP curves. Since the results are the same as shown when R was used, the output is omitted.

```
%cuminc(ds=bmt, time=dftime, cenvble=cens,interest=1,group=tx);
%compcp(ds=follic,time=dftime,cens=cens,group=agecat,val1=0,val2=1);
```

The covariate `agecat` has the value 1 for age greater than 65 and 0 otherwise.

8.2 COMPARING TWO TYPES OF RISK IN THE SAME POPULATION

8.2.1 Theoretical background

Sometimes it is important to know whether in a population some risks are more common than others. For example, in the `follic` dataset it would be of interest to know whether the risk for relapse is larger than the risk of dying of other causes (without relapse).

Chapters 1 and 5 show that, when competing risks are present, comparing the cause-specific hazards between two groups is not equivalent to comparing the subdistribution functions (CIF). However, comparing the cause-specific hazards of two risks of the same population is equivalent to comparing the CIFs. This can be easily seen by writing equation (4.1) for the CIFs of the two risk types:

$$\hat{F}_1(t) = \sum_{\text{all } j,\, t_j \leq t} \hat{h}_{1j}\hat{S}(t_{j-1}) \quad \text{and} \quad \hat{F}_2(t) = \sum_{\text{all } j,\, t_j \leq t} \hat{h}_{2j}\hat{S}(t_{j-1}),$$

where $\hat{S}(t_{j-1})$ is the probability of being free of any event prior to t_j and h_{1j} and h_{2j} are the two types of cause-specific risk. Note that $\hat{S}(t_{j-1})$ is the same in both formulae. Hence comparing h_{1j} with h_{2j} is the same as comparing $\hat{F}_1(t)$ with $\hat{F}_2(t)$.

Kochar *et al.* (2002) discuss the tests available in the literature for comparing the cause-specific hazards for two different types of event. They propose and compare three classes of test statistics. The test based on C_n^* is recommended as being more robust and less sensitive to the type of weight used as compared with the other tests. The class of tests C_n^* is given by

$$C_n^*(w) = \sup_{0 \leq s < t < \infty} \frac{|L_n(t) - L_n(s)|}{\sigma_n}.$$

For the discrete case and the weight given by the number at risk (n_j), $L_n(t)$ is

$$L_n(t) = \sum_{t_j \leq t} \{d_{2j} - d_{1j}\},$$

with d_{1j} and d_{2j} the number of events of type 1 and respectively of type 2 at time t_j. The denominator is given by

$$\sigma_n^2(t) = n \sum_{t_j \leq t} \{d_{2j} + d_{1j}\}.$$

The distribution of $\sqrt{n}C_n^*$ can be approximated by the density

$$f(x) = 8 \sum_{k=1}^{\infty} (-1)^{k-1} k^2 \phi(kx),$$

where ϕ is the density function of the standard normal distribution. Details of this distribution can be found in Feller (1951).

Note that C_n^* tests whether the largest difference between the two CIFs is significantly different from zero.

8.2.2   Using R

The function `kly` given in Appendix B computes the C_n^* statistics and the p-value. The program expects the two types of events to be coded as 1 and 2. For example, to compare the incidence of relapse with the incidence of dying without relapse in the `follic` dataset, relapse can be coded as 1 and death without relapse as 2.

```
> kly(follic$dftime,cens)
     cnw          pvalue
  9.863435   p-value<0.00001
```

The significant p-value suggests that there is a difference between the incidence of relapse and the incidence of dying without relapse. In Figure 8.4 the CIF for relapse is well above the CIF for death without relapse, suppporting the conclusion found using the `kly` function.

8.2.3   Discussion

Suppose that a group of mice are observed until they die, and their times and causes of death are recorded. The causes of death are grouped into two categories: heart failure and other causes. It is

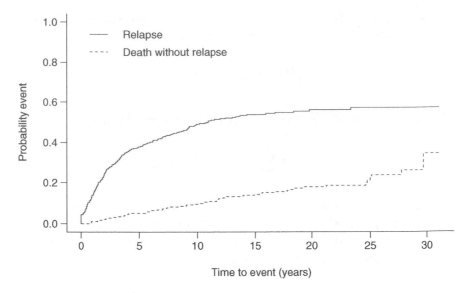

Figure 8.4 Comparing the risk for relapse with the risk for death in the `follic` dataset.

further assumed that the cause-specific hazards for the two types of failure (causes of death) are proportional over time. The follow-up ends only after all the mice have died. Thus all subjects experience a type of failure. The intention is to test whether the risk of death from heart failure exceeds the risk of all the other causes of death. If the risk of death from heart failure is the same as for the other types of failure then it is expected that approximately half of the mice will die of heart failure and the other half will die of other causes. Therefore, the null hypothesis is that the proportion of mice dying of heart failure is half, and the alternative hypothesis is that the proportion is different from 0.5. It is worth mentioning that in this case the time to death does not contain relevant information. Since the two risks are competing, only the time to the first event is observed. If the other causes have a smaller cause-specific hazard than the risk of heart failure, the only observed events of the type 'other' are those few for which the time to event happens to be small.

However, if the cause-specific hazards are not proportional, then testing whether the proportion of deaths from heart failure is different from 0.5 might not be of great interest. It can easily be imagined that if the two CIFs intersect each other the proportion of deaths from hear failure would be approximately the same as the proportion for the other causes of death. The Kochas–Lam–Yip (KLY) test presented in Section 8.2.1 is more powerful. It tests whether at any point in time one curve is significantly higher than the other.

Of crucial importance is the assumption that T, the time to first event, is continuous. Let us apply the KLY test for the data in Table 8.3a:

```
> kly(time,cens)
      cnw       pvalue
  2.121320   0.1353426
```

Table 8.3a Theoretical examples for Kochar, Lam and Yip test.

Time (years)	Type of event*
0.1	1
0.2	1
0.3	1
0.4	1
0.5	1
0.6	1
0.7	1
0.8	1
0.9	1
2.0	1
3.0	2
4.0	1
5.0	2
6.0	1
7.0	2
8.0	1
9.0	2
10.0	1

* 1 = Event of interest, 2 = Competing risk event, 0 = No event.

Table 8.3b Theoretical example for Kochar, Lam and Yip test.

Time (years)	Type of event*
1.0	1
1.0	1
1.0	1
1.0	1
1.0	1
1.0	1
1.0	1
1.0	1
1.0	1
2.0	1
3.0	2
4.0	1
5.0	2
6.0	1
7.0	2
8.0	1
9.0	2
10.0	1

* 1=Event of interest, 2=Competing risk event, 0=No event.

Note that the first nine events are of type 1 and are observed before 1 year. If we approximate these time points to 1 year (Table 8.3b) and we apply the test we obtain a totally different result:

```
> kly(timeappx,cens)
      cnw     pvalue
 0.2357023        1
```

This type of data is usually encountered in cancer research when the event of interest is disease failure at the local site. When a patient does not achieve a complete response after treatment a fixed time for failure is set, usually 1 day. In fact this failure time can be anywhere between 0 and the time after treatment when the response is evaluated (e.g. 3 months).

8.3 IDENTIFIABILITY AND TESTING INDEPENDENCE

As seen in Chapter 3, the concept of competing risks can be defined mathematically in two ways: either as a bivariate distribution (T, C), where T is the time to an event and C is the type of event, or as latent failure times, where the observed time T is the minimum of p possible observable hypothetical times, $T = \min(T_1, T_2, \ldots, T_p)$. The latter definition has a major drawback: the non-identifiability. If only the first event is observed there are many sets of joint distributions $(T_1, T_2, \ldots, T_p)$ which can produce the same marginal distributions. Therefore, in general terms the dependence between the marginal distributions cannot be tested. In the special case where the time to event is purely discrete it was shown (Crowder, 1996, 1997) that a test for independence between the risks can be developed. Crowder's test for independence (Crowder, 1997) can be applied only when many events of each type, including a combination of the events of interest, can be observed at each point in time.

Suppose that it is desired to test whether severe fatigue and gastrointestinal (GI) toxicity (nausea and vomiting) are dependent in a group of patients treated with chemotherapy. The patients are interviewed every week during the 6 months of treatment. Only the first event is recorded since severe toxicity would lead to a change in treatment and the toxicity observed after that would be irrelevant. The first event could be fatigue, GI toxicity or both. The test is based on a function of the subhazard:

$$g_c\left(t_j\right) = \frac{h_c\left(t_j\right)}{1 - h\left(t_j\right)},$$

where $h_c\left(t_j\right)$ is the subhazard for condition c at time t_j and $h\left(t_j\right)$ is the hazard for any condition to be observed at time t_j. The test compares the function g calculated for the combined conditions with the product of between functions g calculated for the individual components. For example, using the subscript f for fatigue, v for GI toxicity and fv for both, the equality which is tested is:

$$g_{fv}\left(t_j\right) = g_f\left(t_j\right) g_v\left(t_j\right).$$

Although the functions g are not probabilities, this equality seems natural for testing independence and Crowder (1996) proved it to be necessary and sufficient for independence.

Ultimately, the test follows a χ^2_{dm} distribution, where dm is the number of degrees of freedom, m being the number of distinct times for which events were observed and d depending on the number of conditions for which the dependence is tested. For example, for p conditions, then

$$d = 2^p - 1 - p.$$

Dewan *et al.* (2004) introduced a test for independence based on the survivor functions rather than the hazard functions. Since the problem of non-identifiability does not arise in this circumstance, the test is more general, encompassing the continuous-time failure situation. This test is based on the conditional probability

$$P(C = i | T < t) = \frac{F_i(t)}{F(t)},$$

where $F_i(t)$ is the CIF for event of type i and $F(t) = P(T < t)$. The test is presented only for two types of events and does not allow censoring. The authors acknowledge these limitations and anticipate new developments in the near future.

8.4   PARAMETRIC MODELLING

8.4.1   Introduction

The mathematical formulation of competing risks (Chapter 3) can be expressed in two ways. For the latent failure time approach, the observed time is the minimum of a collection of random variables representing possible failure times. Alternatively, the competing risks can also be modelled using a bivariate distribution where the first random variable is the observed time and the second indicates the type of event observed. Previous chapters showed how to model in the semiparametric context (proportional hazards). The availability of software made this approach appealing. In contrast, for parametric modelling there is little software available: only the marginal distribution can be modelled. This corresponds to the scenario where the competing risks are ignored. Hence, the interpretation of the analysis is the same as in the case of modelling cause-specific hazards (Chapters 4 and 5). However, knowing the parameters, one can obtain the fitted CIFs for a set of covariates. The estimation of the CIFs assumes, unfortunately, that the different types of events are independent (see the discussion on non-identifiability in Section 3.3.3). In Section A.4 the equations for the latent failure exponential model are derived using the maximum likelihood method. The equations are the same as for the marginal distribution when the competing risks are ignored.

8.4.2 Modelling the marginal distribution

When the marginal distribution is modelled, the competing risks are ignored, and therefore the functions and procedures available in R or SAS can be used. The Weibull distribution is used here an example. A way to estimate the form of the CIF parametrically under the restriction of independence is also shown. For more coverage of parametric modelling for time-to-event analysis, see Lawless (1982) or Collett (2003).

In Chapter 3 the Weibull survivor function was defined as

$$S(t) = \exp\{-(\lambda t)^{\alpha}\}.$$

For the purpose of modelling let us rewrite this as

$$S(t|x) = \exp\left\{-\left(\frac{t}{\theta(x)}\right)^{\alpha}\right\},$$

where α is a shape parameter and θ is a scale parameter which is modelled as a function of the covariates: $\theta(x) = \exp(\beta_0 + \beta_1 x)$. Note that since α is not a function of x, the model still assumes proportionality of hazards. When $\alpha = 1$ the special case of the exponential distribution is obtained.

The parameters are estimated using the maximum likelihood approach. To obtain the parameters the first derivative of the likelihood with respect to each parameter is set equal to zero. A numerical method must be used to solve these equations, since in general they do not have a closed form. Since the approach is essentially the same regardless of the statistical software used, the theory is exemplified using R on a real-life example.

8.4.3   Modelling the Weibull distribution

In this section the time to second malignancy for a group of cancer patients is modelled using the hd dataset (Section 1.6.5), which is a cohort of 865 early stage Hodgkin's disease patients. The aim is to estimate the probability of second malignancy using the Weibull distribution. Death without a second malignancy constitutes the competing risk.

A Weibull distribution is fitted to the marginal distribution for the second malignancy:

```
> fit
Call:
survreg(formula = Surv(maltime, evcens) ~ 1, data = hd)

Coefficients:
(Intercept)
  3.674971

Scale= 0.3911653

Loglik(model)= -668.1  Loglik(intercept only)= -668.1
n= 865
```

and to the marginal distribution for the competing risks:

```
> fit
Call:
survreg(formula = Surv(maltime, crcens) ~ 1, data = hd)

Coefficients:
(Intercept)
  4.209682

Scale= 1.249816
```

```
Loglik(model)= -1298   Loglik(intercept only)= -1298
n= 865
```

Note that the model scale parameters for the event of interest and for competing risks are different (0.391 for second malignancy and 1.249 for the competing risks). Thus, the formula from Table 3.3 cannot be used to write the CIF. However, the subdensity for second malignancy can be written as

$$f_{ev}(t) = \lambda_{ev}\alpha_{ev}(\lambda_{ev}t)^{\alpha_{ev}-1} e^{-\{(\lambda_{ev}t)^{\alpha_{ev}}+(\lambda_{cr}t)^{\alpha_{cr}}\}},$$

where $\lambda_{ev} = 1/\exp(3.675), \lambda_{cr} = 1/\exp(4.21), \alpha_{ev} = 1/0.391$ and $\alpha_{cr} = 1/1.25$. The CIF is

$$F_{ev}(t) = \int_0^t f_{ev}(u)\,du$$

which can be approximated using the trapezoidal rule. Figure 8.5 illustrates the approximation of the CIF based on nonparametric

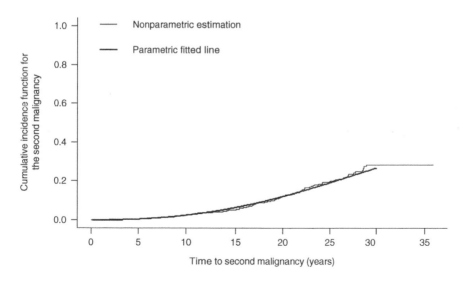

Figure 8.5 Cumulative incidence function of the probability of second malignancy in the hd dataset using the Weibull distribution.

estimation (the step function) and on the estimation of the Weibull distribution (the smooth line).

As mentioned before, the estimation of the CIF using parametric distributions assumes that the event of interest and the competing risk event are independent. This represents a serious limitation of parametric modelling. The reader can consult Larson and Dinse (1985) and Maller and Zhou (2002) for further development of more general models in this framework.

9

Food for thought

The examples in this chapter are intended to provide a deeper understanding of the issues of competing risks, highlighting some of the issues that have been introduced in this book. They are presented in a question–answer style, but the reader may choose not to solve them as exercises.

PROBLEM 1: ESTIMATION OF THE PROBABILITY OF THE EVENT OF INTEREST

The hd dataset (Section 1.6.5) contains the records for 865 Hodgkin's disease patients. There are three types of events: relapse, second malignancy after the diagnosis of Hodgkin's disease, and death. The event of interest is second malignancy. Relapse was observed regardless of whether a second malignancy occurred. If it is assumed that the occurrence of relapse does not alter the probability of a second malignancy, then second malignancy and relapse are not competing events.

(a) Using this dataset, create a variable for time to second malignancy such that relapse and death constitute competing risks.

Competing Risks: A Practical Perspective   M. Pintilie
© 2006 John Wiley & Sons, Ltd

(b) Using the data created in (a), estimate the cumulative incidence function (see Chapter 4) and the complement of the Kaplan–Meier function $(1 - KM)$ for second malignancy. Graph the two curves. Which estimate is larger?

(c) Estimate $1 - KM$ using the time to second malignancy (maltime) and the indicator variable (mcens) as given in the hd dataset. Add the line defined by these estimates to the plot obtained in part (b). Which of the two initial curves is closer to the newly added curve? Why?

(d) Graph the CIF for the original data (maltime, mcens) considering death as the only competing risk.

Solution

(a) If for each patient only the first event is observed, then second malignancy and relapse are competing events. To create the time variable the R command is

```
> alltime=apply(cbind(hd$dftime,hd$maltime),1,min)
```

where hd$dftime is time to relapse or death and hd$maltime is time to second malignancy. In this way, alltime is the time at which the first event was observed: relapse, second malignancy or death. A censoring variable can be generated using the censoring variable for relapse and death, hd$dfcens, and the censoring variable for the second malignancy, hd$mcens:

```
> allcens=apply(cbind(hd$dfcens,hd$mcens),1,max)
```

Thus, allcens takes the value 1 if any of the above events were observed and 0 otherwise. Two indicator variables are created: one for second malignancy as the first event and another for competing risks:

```
mlcens=(alltime==hd$maltime & hd$mcens==1)+0
crlcens=(alltime==hd$dftime & hd$dfcens==1)+0
```

The censoring variable for the competing risks situation is:

```
cens=mlcens+2*crlcens
```

(b) The graph for the CIF can be created with the commands:

```
> fitcr=cuminc(alltime,cens)
> forplot=list(list(fitcr$'1 1'$time,fitcr$'11'$est))
> plot.cuminc(forplot)
```

The line for $1 - KM$ can be added to it:

```
> fitcs1=survfit(Surv(alltime,m1cens)~ 1)
> lines(fitcs1,fun='event',lty=2)
```

The $1 - KM$ estimates are larger because they ignore the competing risks. More details on this topic can be found in Chapters 1 and 4.

(c) We can add the $1 - KM$ estimates for the original data, when second malignancy was observed regardless of the time it occurred, either before or after relapse:

```
> fitcs2=survfit(Surv(maltime,mcens)~1,data=hd)
> lines(fitcs2,fun='event',lty=3)
```

The line for $1 - KM$ estimates for the original data falls very close to the $1 - KM$ estimated for the second malignancy as the first event. The estimates given by $1 - KM$ ignore the competing risks. The curve represents the exponential of the cumulative cause-specific hazard. Whether it is estimated when the competing risks are relapse and death or the competing risks are only the deaths, the curve is about the same. On the other hand, the CIF depends on what competing risks are considered.

(d) The CIF when death is the only competing risk can be added to the existing graph:

```
> cens=hd$mcens+2*(hd$mcens==0 & hd$stat==1)
> fitcr=cuminc(hd$maltime,cens)
> lines(fitcr$'1 1'$time,fitcr$'1 1'$est,lty=4)
```

This curve is between the $1 - KM$ estimates which ignore all competing risks and the CIF when relapse and death are competing risks.

Figure 9.1 illustrates these four curves.

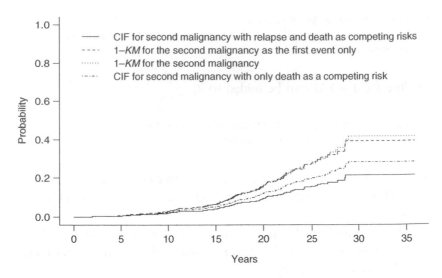

Figure 9.1 Curves for second malignancy in the hd dataset.

The focus of this problem is the estimation of the probability of an event and its relationship with the $1 - KM$ estimate. The higher the incidence of the competing risks, the further the $1 - KM$ estimate is from the probability of an event.

PROBLEM 2: TESTING A COVARIATE

The tamrt dataset (Section 1.6.1) contains information on a group of early stage breast cancer patients randomized to tamoxifen alone (Tam) or radiation and tamoxifen (RT+Tam). The intention is to test the effect of the treatment (tx) on local relapse. Compare the results obtained using Gray's test (Chapter 5) and the log-rank test. Justify your answer.

Solution

To carry out Gray's test the cuminc function is applied. The censoring variable needs to be created. The R commands are:

```
> cens=tamrt$lcens+2*(tamrt$lcens==0 & tamrt$stat==1)
```

The test results are:

```
> cuminc(tamrt$loctime,cens,tamrt$tx)
Tests:
```

	stat	pv	df
1	**28.014443**	**1.204134e-07**	1
2	2.858190	9.090977e-02	1

The estimates of the probability of local relapse and their variance are given below. The first two lines refer to the event of interest for the two groups, marked as 'B 1' and 'T 1', and next two lines refer to the competing risks ('B 2' and 'T 2').

```
$est
```

		2	4	6	8
B	1	0.003144716	0.003144716	0.003144716	0.03506651
T	1	0.041125927	0.075168127	0.104514279	0.18616441
B	2	0.037912666	0.065755626	0.076171109	0.10359779
T	2	0.015828494	0.040081620	0.054890682	0.06914639

```
$var
```

		2	4	6	8
B	1	9.889736e-06	9.889736e-06	9.889736e-06	0.0003968316
T	1	1.251715e-04	2.288378e-04	3.559369e-04	0.0015799465
B	2	1.156354e-04	2.037439e-04	2.558497e-04	0.0004899353
T	2	4.948572e-05	1.294571e-04	1.980208e-04	0.0003954587

The χ^2 with 1 degree of freedom for Gray's test is 28.014.

The results for log-rank test can be obtained as follows:

```
> survdiff(Surv(loctime,lcens)~tx,data=tamrt)
Call:
survdiff(formula = Surv(loctime, lcens) ~ tx, data = tamrt)
```

	N	Observed	Expected	(O-E)^2/E	(O-E)^2/V
tx=B	320	4	20.3	13.1	27.4
tx=T	321	35	18.7	14.2	27.4

Chisq= 27.4 on 1 degrees of freedom, p= 1.63e-07

The results are about the same (χ^2 with 1 degree of freedom is 27.4) for the logrank test) because the study is randomized and the treatment is not expected to change the competing risks (here, death without local relapse).

PROBLEM 3: COMPARING THE EVENT OF INTEREST BETWEEN TWO GROUPS WHEN THE COMPETING RISKS ARE DIFFERENT FOR EACH GROUP

As in Problem 1, a competing risks situation can be created in the hd dataset (Section 1.6.5) by considering only the first event observed. The event of interest is second malignancy (the first malignancy after diagnosis of Hodgkin's disease) and the competing risk is the observation of either relapse or death. Dichotomize the age variable: 0 for age < 30 and 1 otherwise. Test this variable either using the crr function and thus taking into account the competing risks, or using the coxph function where the competing risks are ignored. Test the dichotomized variable for age as described below:

A. Apply the crr function with second malignancy as the event of interest and using both relapse and death as competing risks.
B. Apply the coxph function with second malignancy as the event of interest and using both relapse and death as competing risks.
C. Apply the crr function with second malignancy as the event of interest using only death as the competing risk.
D. Apply the coxph function with second malignancy as the event of interest and using only death as the competing risk.

Each model produces a coefficient, representing the effect of age on the second malignancy under different conditions. Which coefficient is larger? Why?

Solution

Note that for models A and B the time to first event is defined in the same way as in Problem 1, while for models C and D the time to second malignancy is defined as in the hd dataset.

Each type of model (hazard of subdistribution or cause-specific hazard) gives some information on the effect of the covariate. Models B and D give the 'ideal effect', the effect that could have been observed if the competing risks did not exist (Figure 9.2, top). Thus for models

Models B and D: Competing risks are ignored

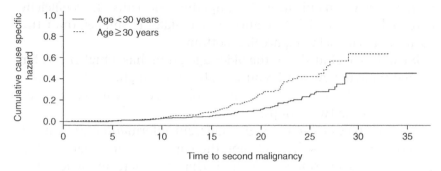

Time to second malignancy

Model A: Relaspe and death are competing risks

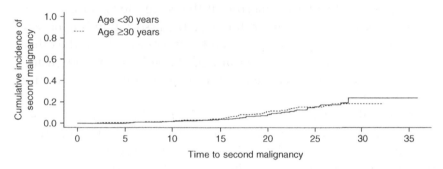

Time to second malignancy

Model C: Only death is competing risk

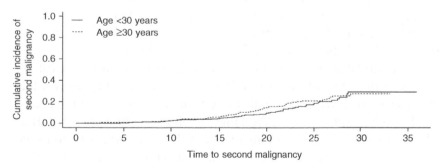

Time to second malignancy

Figure 9.2 The effect of age under the different models.

B and D the coefficients are similar and larger than for both models
A and C. The effects seen in models A and C are the 'real effects'.
Model A gives the effect of age on second malignancy when only
the first event was observed. The events that form the competing

risks are relapse and death. Model C gives the effect of age on second malignancy when only death is competing risk. Thus, the coefficient obtained using model A (Figure 9.2, middle) is smaller than the coefficient of model C (Figure 9.2, bottom).

It can be concluded that the older age group has a higher risk for second malignancy, but because it also has a higher risk for other conditions (relapse and/or death) the observed prevalence is about the same in the two groups.

The two types of analysis give different information and thus it is necessary to do both. Modelling the cause-specific hazard (using coxph) gives information on how that covariate influences the outcome in a 'laboratory' setting where competing risks do not exist. This could be very important if the covariate is, for example, a genetic or biological marker. If indeed the association is apparent then a biological or genetic path can be hypothesized. On the other hand, the modelling of the hazard of the subdistribution (using crr) gives the real effect seen in the dataset under study or in a similar dataset.

Suppose that a treatment has a significant effect when the cause-specific hazard is tested but the effect is minimal when the hazard of the subdistribution is modelled. In this case it can be concluded that the treatment has an effect at the biological level. However, in the population in which it was tested there was no real effect, possibly due to an increase in the competing risks. Further investigations could reveal that the treatment was very aggressive and caused severe side effects. Thus a weaker dose could be tried.

A similar situation may occur when a biological marker is tested. Suppose that patients with positive markers have a higher risk for relapse as well as for second malignancy. If only the first event (either relapse or second malignancy) is observed, and provided that there are enough observations to detect the difference, the analysis of cause-specific hazard will be significant while the analysis of the hazard of the subdistribution will not.

The actual R code and the results follow. In preparation for applying the models the time to first event and its censoring variable are created:

```
> alltime=apply(cbind(hd$dftime,hd$maltime),1,min)
> allcens=apply(cbind(hd$dfcens,hd$mcens),1,max)
```

Also required are the censoring variable for second malignancy as the first event (m1cens) and the censoring variables for the crr function for model A (cens1) and for model C (cens2):

```
> m1cens=(alltime==hd$maltime & hd$mcens==1)+0
> cr1cens=(alltime==hd$dftime & hd$dfcens==1)+0
> cens1=m1cens+2*cr1cens
> cens2=hd$mcens+2*(hd$mcens==0 & hd$stat==1)
```

The variable to be tested is

```
x=(hd$age>=30)+0
```

The models can now be applied in two. First, model A:

```
> crr(alltime,cens1,x)
convergence: TRUE
coefficients:
[1] 0.06075
standard errors:
[1] 0.2044
two-sided p-values:
[1] 0.77
```

Next, model B:

```
> coxph(Surv(alltime,m1cens) ~ x)
Call:
coxph(formula = Surv(alltime, m1cens) ~ x)

      coef   exp(coef)   se(coef)      z      p
x   0.437        1.55      0.210   2.08  0.037
Likelihood ratio test=4.17 on 1 df, p=0.0412 n= 860
```

Third, model C:

```
> crr(hd$maltime,cens2,x)
convergence: TRUE
coefficients:
[1] 0.1726
standard errors:
[1] 0.175
two-sided p-values:
[1] 0.32
```

Finally, model D:

```
> coxph(Surv(maltime,mcens) ~ x,data=hd)
Call:
coxph(formula = Surv(maltime, mcens) ~ x, data = hd)
```

```
       coef    exp(coef)    se(coef)      z        p
x     0.569        1.77       0.180    3.17   0.0015
```

Likelihood ratio test=10.1 on 1 df, p=0.00145 n= 865

To summarize, the coefficients for the four models are: A, 0.060 75; B, 0.437; C, 0.1726; D, 0.569.

This example illustrates the fact that the modelling of the cause-specific hazard is invariant to the competing risks existing in the dataset. The generalization of the modelling of the hazard of the subdistribution is limited to datasets of the same type – with the same competing risks.

PROBLEM 4: INFORMATION NEEDED FOR SAMPLE SIZE CALCULATIONS

A new treatment, successful in a phase II trial, is believed to improve the local relapse rate in patients diagnosed with follicular lymphoma. A randomized study needs to be designed to support this hypothesis. What information does one need to calculate the sample size necessary to detect a clinical significant difference between the local relapse incidence in the standard treatment and in the experimental treatment? How does the sample size change if the population eligible for the study is young or old?

Solution

Apart from the usual information on the type I and II error (α and β), we need to know the incidence of local relapse at a certain point in time and the clinically significant difference that needs to be detected. It is necessary to clarify what are the competing risks and their incidence in each arm. If local relapse is observed regardless of the observation of other relapses then only death is a competing risk. However, it is very likely that the rate of local relapse changes after another type of relapse is observed. This is due to the fact that, for the observed relapse, the patient receives some treatment which influences the rate of local relapse. Thus, it is more accurate to assume that any other type of relapse is also a competing risk.

One has to specify whether the effect size is in terms of the hazard of the subdistribution or the cause-specific hazard.

It is to be expected that if the study is carried out on an elderly population there will be more competing risks and therefore fewer events of interest will be observed. Thus a larger sample size is needed when the population is old than when it is young. The power can be calculated using the R function `power` given in Appendix B.

PROBLEM 5: THE EFFECT OF THE SIZE OF THE INCIDENCE OF COMPETING RISKS ON THE COEFFICIENT OBTAINED IN THE MODEL

A randomized study is carried out to test the effect of the experimental treatment on relapse. Suppose that the experimental treatment lowers the incidence of relapse as well as the incidence of competing risks. How would the test for the hazard of the subdistribution (using the `crr` function, for example) differ from the test for the cause-specific hazard (using the `coxph` function)? Simulate two datasets to exemplify this above problem: one for which the competing risks are not affected by the experimental treatment, and one for which they are.

Solution

Since the experimental treatment affects both the relapse incidence and the competing risks, it is likely that in the experimental treatment we will observe more relapses than we would have observed had we had the same competing risks as in the standard arm. Thus, the difference between the two arms when the hazard of the subdistribution is modelled will appear smaller than when the cause-specific hazard is modelled.

A simulation of a dataset for which the competing risks are affected by the experimental treatment is shown below. The case where they are not, can be similarly obtained by making the cause-specific hazard for the competing risks for the experimental arm equal to the cause-specific hazard in the standard arm.

Suppose that the cause-specific hazard in the standard arm for relapse is 0.2 and for competing risks is 0.4. Each of these is affected by the experimental treatment, becoming respectively 0.1 and 0.2. Suppose that 400 patients are accrued in each arm. Assume that the accrual is uniform over a period of 5 years and that 2 extra years are added to the follow-up. The treatment is coded as 1 for the standard arm and 0 for the experimental arm.

The R commands are:

```
> a=5
> f=2
> levs=.2
> lcrs=.4
> leve=.1
> lcre=.2
> n=400
> x=rep(c(1,0),each=n)
> t0=rep(c(1:n)/n*a+f,2)
> set.seed(1)  ## for reproducibility
> tev=c(rexp(n,levs),rexp(n,leve))
> tcr=c(rexp(n,lcrs),rexp(n,lcre))
> time=apply(cbind(t0,tev,tcr),1,min)
> ev=(tev==time)+0
> cr=(tcr==time)+0
> cens=ev+2*(ev==0 & cr==1)
```

The model for the hazard of the subdistribution gives:

```
> crr(time,cens,x)
convergence: TRUE
coefficients:
[1] 0.3917
standard errors:
[1] 0.135
two-sided p-values:
[1] 0.0037
```

Modelling the cause-specific hazard gives:

```
> coxph(Surv(time,ev) ~ x)
Call:
coxph(formula = Surv(time, ev) ~ x)
```

```
      coef exp(coef) se(coef)     z        p
x 0.742       2.1    0.139 5.35 8.8e-08
Likelihood ratio test=29.2 on 1 df, p=6.61e-08 n= 800
```

If the competing risks are ignored, the theoretical effect size as given by the hazard ratio is `levs/leve` $= 0.2/0.1 = 2$.

The coefficient for the cause-specific hazard model is 0.742 and the hazard ratio is 2.1. The coefficient for the hazard of the subdistribution modelling is considerably less, at 0.392. When competing risks are ignored the rate of event of interest in the standard arm is larger than in the experimental arm. Accounting for the competing risks makes the difference between the two arms smaller because more of the events of interest in the standard arm are not observed than in the experimental arm.

PROBLEM 6: THE KLY TEST AND THE NON-PROPORTIONALITY OF HAZARDS

Apply the Kochar–Lam–Yip test introduced in Section 8.2 to the `hd` dataset (section 1.6.5). Assume that the event of interest is death due to Hodgkin's disease (indicator variable `cscens`) and that the competing risks are all other causes. Draw the CIF for the two types of events. Discuss the results.

Solution

Let us create the censoring variable,

```
>cens=hd$cscens+2*(hd$cscens==0 & hd$stat==1)
```

and apply the test using the `kly` function given in the Appendix B:

```
> kly(hd$survtime,cens)
     cnw            pvalue
7.121806  p-value<0.00001
```

The test gives a highly statistically significant *p*-value. The CIF curves are drawn in Figure 9.3 using the commands:

```
> fit=cuminc(hd$survtime,cens)
> plot.cuminc(fit, curvlab=c("Death due to Hodgkin's Disease",
      "Death due to other causes"))
```

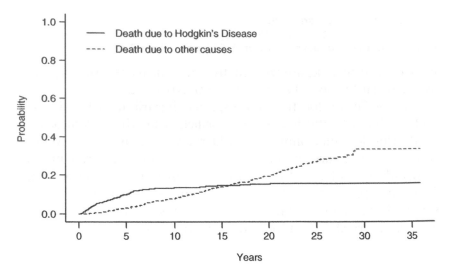

Figure 9.3 The cumulative incidence functions for death due to Hodgkin's disease and other causes.

The KLY test looks for the largest difference at any point in time. Thus the significance is not influenced by the fact that the two curves intersect but by the fact that either between 5 and 10 years or somewhere after 25 years the two curves are sufficiently far apart.

PROBLEM 7: THE KLY AND WILCOXON TESTS

Compare the CIF for second malignancy and the CIF for death without second malignancy in the tamrt dataset (Section 1.6.1). Consider only the subset of those with events. First, apply the KLY test. Compare also the time to second malignancy with the time to death without second malignancy using the Wilcoxon rank-sum test. Calculate the means and medians for the time to second malignancy and for the time to death without second malignancy. Simulate a dataset for which the time to event and time to competing risks follow exponential distributions. Repeat the above analysis. Discuss the results.

Solution

As before, the proper censoring variable is first created:

```
> cens=tamrt$mcens+2*(tamrt$mcens==0 & tamrt$stat==1)
```

Let us take the subset of those with events. Note that this is not a requirement of the KLY test but rather a condition imposed here to illustrate the connection between the KLY and Wilcoxon tests.

```
> time=tamrt$maltime[cens>0]
> cens2=cens[cens >0]
```

Applying the KLY test, a statistically significant *p*-value is obtained (Figure 9.4):

```
> kly(time,cens2)
     cnw         pvalue
3.197406    0.005545024
```

Since in this subset for each patient an event was observed and thus we do not have censoring, it is tempting to apply the Wilcoxon rank-sum test to compare the time to second malignancy with the time to death without second malignancy.

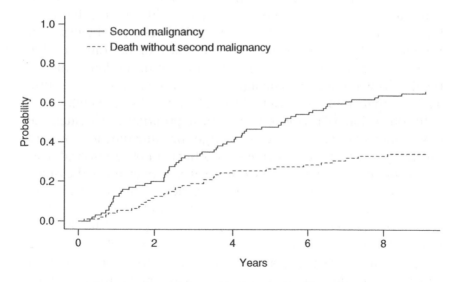

Figure 9.4 Cumulative incidence function for the second malignancy and death without second malignancy in the `tamrt` dataset.

```
> t1=time[cens2==1]
> t2=time[cens2==2]
> wilcox.test(t1,t2)
        Wilcoxon rank sum test with continuity correction
data: t1 and t2 W = 1047,    p-value = 0.6637 alternative
hypothesis:true mu is not equal to 0
```

The *p*-value for the Wilcoxon test is not statistically significant. This is not a mere expression of type II error. The means and medians of the two time variables are found to be similar:

```
> by(time,cens2,mean)
INDICES: 1
[1] 3.448014
INDICES: 2
[1] 3.222194
> by(time,cens2,median)
INDICES: 1
[1] 2.977413
INDICES: 2
[1] 2.632444
```

The two results are not contradictory. The KLY test tests whether there is a difference large enough at some point in time, while the Wilcoxon rank-sum test compares the centre of the two distributions. Figure 9.4 is in agreement with the KLY test. As discussed in Section 8.2.3, second malignancy occurs at a higher rate but, due to the fact that only the first event is observed, the long time for the deaths without second malignancy cannot be observed because a second malignancy beats it to the mark and is observed first.

In conclusion, Wilcoxon test is not the appropriate test because the observation of the time to second malignancy and time to death are not independent: if one is observed, the other cannot be observed. This is true for any test applied to the time to event, for example the *t*-test.

To simulate such an example, let us generate time to event from an exponential distribution of hazard of 0.2 and time to competing risks from an exponential distribution of hazard of 0.1. The observed time is the minimum of the two time variables and a censoring variable can be created appropriately: 1 when the event of interest was observed (time to event of interest was smaller than the time to competing risks) and 2 otherwise. The simulation is similar to what was shown in Problem 5 and the details are omitted.

Appendix A
Theoretical background

A.1 NONPARAMETRIC MAXIMUM LIKELIHOOD ESTIMATION FOR THE SURVIVOR FUNCTION IN THE DISCRETE CASE

Let $t_1, t_2, \ldots, t_r$ be the unique failure time points with $t_1 < t_2 < \ldots < t_r$. Denote by d_j the number of failures, n_j the number at risk and at time t_j, and m_j the number of individuals censored in the interval $[t_{j-1}, t_j)$. Then the likelihood function can be written as

$$L = \prod_{j=1}^{r} \left[S\left(t_{j-1}\right) - S\left(t_j\right) \right]^{d_j} S\left(t_{j-1}\right)^{m_j}.$$

Replacing S(t) with the expression in (2.5), where the notation $h_j = h\left(t_j\right)$ is implied, and working through the algebra leads to the following simplification:

$$L = \prod_{j=1}^{r} \left\{ \left[\prod_{i=1}^{j-1}(1 - h_i) - \prod_{i=1}^{j}(1 - h_i) \right]^{d_j} \left[\prod_{i=1}^{j-1}(1 - h_i) \right]^{m_j} \right\}$$

Competing Risks: A Practical Perspective   M. Pintilie
© 2006 John Wiley & Sons, Ltd

$$
= \prod_{j=1}^{r} \left\{ \left[\prod_{i=1}^{j-1} (1-h_i) \right]^{d_j} \left[1-1+h_j \right]^{d_j} \left[\prod_{i=1}^{j-1} (1-h_i) \right]^{m_j} \right\}
$$

$$
= \prod_{j=1}^{r} \left\{ h_j^{d_j} \left[\prod_{i=1}^{j-1} (1-h_i) \right]^{d_j+m_j} \right\}
$$

$$
= \left\{ \prod_{j=1}^{r} h_j^{d_j} \right\} \left\{ \prod_{j=1}^{r} \prod_{i=1}^{j-1} (1-h_i)^{d_j+m_j} \right\}
$$

$$
= \left\{ \prod_{j=1}^{r} h_j^{d_j} \right\} \left\{ \prod_{i=1}^{r} \prod_{j=i+1}^{r} (1-h_i)^{d_j+m_j} \right\}
$$

$$
= \left\{ \prod_{j=1}^{r} h_j^{d_j} \right\} \left\{ \prod_{i=1}^{r} (1-h_i)^{\sum_{j=i+1}^{r} (d_j+m_j)} \right\}
$$

$$
= \left\{ \prod_{j=1}^{r} h_j^{d_j} \right\} \left\{ \prod_{i=1}^{r} (1-h_i)^{n_i-d_i} \right\}
$$

$$
= \prod_{j=1}^{r} h_j^{d_j} (1-h_j)^{n_j-d_j}.
$$

Taking logarithms and differentiating with respect to h_j gives

$$
\frac{\partial \log L}{\partial h_j} = \frac{d_j}{h_j} - \frac{n_j - d_j}{1 - h_j}.
$$

Setting this equation to 0, the estimate of h_j is

$$
\hat{h}_j = \frac{d_j}{n_j}.
$$

The formula for the product-limit estimator is obtained when this quantity is substituted into (2.5):

$$
\hat{S}(t) = \prod_{t_j \leq t} \left\{ 1 - \frac{d_j}{n_j} \right\} = \prod_{t_j \leq t} \left\{ \frac{n_j - d_j}{n_j} \right\}.
$$

A.2 CONFIDENCE INTERVAL FOR SURVIVOR FUNCTION

To avoid having confidence interval limits outside the interval $[0, 1]$, Kalbfleisch and Prentice (1980) proposed $\log(-\log)$-transforming the survival estimate, constructing the confidence interval on the resulting quantity and transforming the interval back to the original scale.

Let $T = \log\left(-\log\left(\hat{S}\right)\right)$. The variance of T can be calculated by applying the delta method twice:

$$\text{Var}\left(T\right) = \left(\frac{1}{\log\left(\hat{S}\right)}\right)^2 \text{Var}\left(\log\left(\hat{S}\right)\right)$$

$$= \left(\frac{1}{\log\left(\hat{S}\right)}\right)^2 \left(\frac{1}{\hat{S}}\right)^2 \text{Var}\left(\hat{S}\right)$$

$$= \frac{\text{Var}\left(\hat{S}\right)}{\left(\hat{S}\log\left(\hat{S}\right)\right)^2}.$$

Denote by (T_l, T_u) the confidence interval for T and (S_l, S_u) the confidence interval for $\hat{S}$. The upper bound is derived as follows:

$$T_u = T + z_{1-\alpha/2}\sqrt{\text{Var}\left(T\right)}$$

$$\log\left(-\log\left(S_u\right)\right) = \log\left(-\log\left(\hat{S}\right)\right) + z_{1-\alpha/2}\sqrt{\text{Var}\left(T\right)}$$

$$-\log\left(S_u\right) = -\log\left(\hat{S}\right) e^{z_{1-\alpha/2}\sqrt{\text{Var}(T)}}$$

$$S_u = \hat{S}^{\exp\left(z_{1-\alpha/2}\sqrt{\text{Var}(T)}\right)}.$$

A.3   THE VARIANCE FOR GRAY'S TEST

These are the formulae for the variance for the test statistics given in Section 5.2.1 for the discrete case and two groups. The usual notation is employed: for $i = 1$, 2, let $t_1, t_2, t_3, \ldots, t_j, \ldots, t_n$ be the unique ordered time points at which any type of event happened; $d_i(t)$ the number of events of interest in group i at time t; $c_i(t)$ the number of competing risks type of events in group i at time t; $n_i(t)$ the number at risk in group i at time t; $F_i(t)$ the cumulative incidence probability of the event of interest for group i at time t; and $S_i(t)$ the Kaplan–Meier estimate for the survivor function when all types of events are considered for group i at time t. Then

$$F^0(t_j) = \sum_{i=1}^{j} \frac{d_1(t_j) + d_2(t_j)}{m_1(t_j) + m_2(t_j)}$$

where

$$m_i(t_j) = \frac{n_i(t_j)}{S_i(t_{j-1})}.$$

Since all the formulae below are calculated at a time point t, the time point is suppressed. When the calculation is performed at a previous time point t_{j-1} an underscore (_) is added to the right of the quantity. The indices 1 and 2 refer to the group, and when the quantity is calculated for both groups an index i is used:

$$A = \frac{m_1 m_2}{m_1 + m_2},$$

$$C = \sum_{\text{all } t_j < t} A \frac{d_1 + d_2}{(m_1 + m_2)(1 - F_-^0)},$$

$$\tilde{C} = \sum_{\text{all } t_j} A \frac{d_1 + d_2}{(m_1 + m_2)(1 - F_-^0)}.$$

For each group and for each time t at which an event of interest occurred:

$$tev4_i = 1 - \frac{1 - F^0}{S_i},$$

$$tev3_i = (d_1 + d_2) \frac{S_{i,-}}{(m_1 + m_2) n_i} \left(1 - \frac{d_1 + d_2 - 1}{(m_1 + m_2) S_{i,-} - 1}\right),$$

$$tev1_i = (-1)^{i-1} (A - t4_i C).$$

For each group and for each time t at which a competing risk event occurred:

$$tcr4_i = \frac{1 - F^0}{S_i},$$

$$tcr3_i = c_i \frac{S_{i,-}^2}{n_i^2} \left(1 - \frac{d_i - 1}{n_i - 1}\right),$$

$$tcr1_i = (-1)^{i-1} t4_i C,$$

$$v3_i = \sum_{\text{all } t_j} \left\{tev4_i^2 tev3_i + tcr4_i^2 tcr3_i\right\},$$

$$v2_i = \sum_{\text{all } t_j} \left\{tev1_i tev4_i tev3_i + tcr1_i tcr4_i tcr3_i\right\},$$

$$vpart = \sum_{i=1,2} \sum_{\text{all } t_j} \left\{tev1_i^2 tev3_i + tcr1_i^2 tcr3_i\right\}.$$

The variance is then given by

$$V = vpart + \tilde{C}^2 v3_1 + 2\tilde{C} v2_1 + \tilde{C}^2 v3_2 - 2\tilde{C} v2_2.$$

A.4 DERIVATION OF THE PARAMETERS FOR THE EXPONENTIAL LATENT FAILURE TIME MODEL

Let V be the set of cases for which the event of interest was observed, R the set of cases for which a competing risk type of event was observed, and C the set of censored observations. Denote by $t_i, i = 1, \ldots, n$, all the observed time points. Assume the latent failure definition for the competing risks and independence between the event of interest and competing risks. The subdensity function for the event of interest has the form

$$f_{ev}(t) = \lambda_{ev} e^{-(\lambda_{ev} + \lambda_{cr})t},$$

with the subdistribution given by

$$F_{ev}(t) = \frac{\lambda_{ev}}{\lambda_{ev} + \lambda_{cr}} \left(1 - e^{-(\lambda_{ev} + \lambda_{cr})t}\right).$$

The probability of experiencing neither the event of interest nor the competing event is given by

$$S(t) = e^{-(\lambda_{ev} + \lambda_{cr})t}.$$

The likelihood function can be written as

$$L = \prod_{i \in V} \lambda_{ev} e^{-(\lambda_{ev} + \lambda_{cr})t_i} \prod_{i \in R} \lambda_{cr} e^{-(\lambda_{ev} + \lambda_{cr})t_i} \prod_{i \in C} e^{-(\lambda_{ev} + \lambda_{cr})t_i}$$

$$= \prod_{i \in V} \lambda_{ev} \prod_{i \in R} \lambda_{cr} \prod_{i=1}^{n} e^{-(\lambda_{ev} + \lambda_{cr})t_i}.$$

Taking logs:

$$\log(L) = \sum_{i \in V} \log(\lambda_{ev}) + \sum_{i \in R} \log(\lambda_{cr}) - \sum_{i=1}^{n} (\lambda_{ev} + \lambda_{cr}) t_i$$

$$= n_{ev} \log(\lambda_{ev}) + n_{cr} \log(\lambda_{cr}) - (\lambda_{ev} + \lambda_{cr}) \sum_{i=1}^{n} t_i,$$

where n_{ev} and n_{cr} are respectively the observed numbers of events of interest and competing risks events. It is obvious that by differentiating with respect to λ_{ev} and λ_{cr} the same equations are obtained as if the other type of event did not exist:

$$\frac{n_{ev}}{\lambda_{ev}} - \sum_{i=1}^{n} t_i = 0,$$

$$\frac{n_{cr}}{\lambda_{cr}} - \sum_{i=1}^{n} t_i = 0.$$

A.5 LIKELIHOOD OF A MIXTURE OF EXPONENTIALS IN THE BIVARIATE APPROACH

Denote by V the set of observed events of interest, R the set of observed competing risks and by C the set of censored observations. The total number of observations is n and $t_i, i = 1, \ldots, n$, are the observed time points. The subdensity and the subdistribution for the event of interest are:

$$f_{ev}(t) = p_{ev} \lambda_{ev} e^{-\lambda_{ev} t},$$
$$F_{ev}(t) = p_{ev} \left(1 - e^{-\lambda_{ev} t}\right).$$

The corresponding functions for the competing risks are:

$$f_{cr}(t) = p_{cr} \lambda_{cr} e^{-\lambda_{cr} t},$$
$$F_{cr}(t) = p_{cr} \left(1 - e^{\lambda_{cr} t}\right).$$

The probability of not observing a failure is:

$$S(t) = 1 - F_{ev}(t) - F_{cr}(t) = p_{ev} e^{-\lambda_{ev} t} + p_{cr} e^{-\lambda_{cr} t}.$$

Since $S(0) = 1$, it follows that

$$p_{ev} + p_{cr} = 1.$$

The likelihood takes the form

$$L = \prod_{i \in V} p_{ev} \lambda_{ev} e^{-\lambda_{ev} t_i} \prod_{i \in R} p_{cr} \lambda_{cr} e^{-\lambda_{cr} t_i} \prod_{i \in C} \left\{ p_{ev} e^{-\lambda_{ev} t_i} + p_{cr} e^{-\lambda_{cr} t_i} \right\}.$$

Taking logs:

$$\log(L) = n_{ev}\log(p_{ev}) + n_{ev}\log(\lambda_{ev}) - \lambda_{ev}\sum_{i\in V}t_i$$

$$+ n_{cr}\log(p_{cr}) + n_{cr}\log(\lambda_{cr}) - \lambda_{cr}\sum_{i\in R}t_i$$

$$+ \sum_{i\in C}\log\left(p_{ev}e^{-\lambda_{ev}t_i} + p_{cr}e^{-\lambda_{cr}t_i}\right).$$

where n_{ev} and n_{cr} are respectively the observed numbers of events of interest and competing risk events. To obtain the equations, we differentiate with respect to λ_{ev}, λ_{cr} and p_{ev} (note that p_{cr} is uniquely defined by p_{ev}):

$$\frac{\partial\log(L)}{\partial\lambda_{ev}} = \frac{n_{ev}}{\lambda_{ev}} - \sum_{i\in V}t_i - \sum_{i\in C}\frac{p_{ev}t_ie^{-\lambda_{ev}t_i}}{p_{ev}e^{-\lambda_{ev}t_i} + p_{cr}e^{-\lambda_{cr}t_i}},$$

$$\frac{\partial\log(L)}{\partial\lambda_{cr}} = \frac{n_{cr}}{\lambda_{cr}} - \sum_{i\in R}t_i - \sum_{i\in C}\frac{p_{cr}t_ie^{-\lambda_{cr}t_i}}{p_{ev}e^{-\lambda_{ev}t_i} + p_{cr}e^{-\lambda_{cr}t_i}},$$

$$\frac{\partial\log(L)}{\partial p_{ev}} = \frac{n_{ev}}{p_{ev}} - \frac{n_{cr}}{p_{cr}} + \sum_{i\in C}\frac{e^{-\lambda_{ev}t_i} - e^{-\lambda_{cr}t_i}}{p_{ev}e^{-\lambda_{ev}t_i} + p_{cr}e^{-\lambda_{cr}t_i}}.$$

The parameters λ_{ev}, λ_{cr} and p_{ev} can be obtained from:

$$\frac{n_{ev}}{\lambda_{ev}} - \sum_{i\in V}t_i - \sum_{i\in C}\frac{p_{ev}t_ie^{-\lambda_{ev}t_i}}{p_{ev}e^{-\lambda_{ev}t_i} + p_{cr}e^{-\lambda_{cr}t_i}} = 0,$$

$$\frac{n_{cr}}{\lambda_{cr}} - \sum_{i\in R}t_i - \sum_{i\in C}\frac{p_{cr}t_ie^{-\lambda_{cr}t_i}}{p_{ev}e^{-\lambda_{ev}t_i} + p_{cr}e^{-\lambda_{cr}t_i}} = 0,$$

$$\frac{n_{ev}}{p_{ev}} - \frac{n_{cr}}{p_{cr}} + \sum_{i\in C}\frac{e^{-\lambda_{ev}t_i} - e^{-\lambda_{cr}t_i}}{p_{ev}e^{-\lambda_{ev}t_i} + p_{cr}e^{-\lambda_{cr}t_i}} = 0.$$

This system of equations does not have a closed-form solution.

Appendix B

Analysing competing risks data using R and SAS

B.1 THE R SOFTWARE AND cmprsk PACKAGE

R is free statistical software, developed by John Chambers and colleagues at Bell Laboratories. Its syntax is very much like that of S-PLUS, and it can run on UNIX platforms and similar systems (including FreeBSD and Linux) as well as on Windows 9x/NT/2000/XP and MacOS. The main reason for using this software is that it has a package, cmprsk, developed by Robert Gray, which deals with competing risks.

B.1.1 Downloading and installation

R can be downloaded from http://www.r-project.org. Once there, select **CRAN**, and then choose a mirror site at a convenient geographical location. For example, there are two Canadian sites at http://probability.ca/cran and http://cran.stat.sfu.ca, 2 UK sites (http://cran.uk.r-project.org and http://www.sourcekeg.co.uk/cran/) and 11 US locations. Having

Competing Risks: A Practical Perspective   M. Pintilie
© 2006 John Wiley & Sons, Ltd

chosen a suitable site, first select **R Binaries**, followed by the appropriate operating system, and then **Base** to download the R software. Installation instructions can also be accessed from the download page.

There are many available packages that can be downloaded directly from R. Having installed and opened R, select Packages from the menu bar, then Set CRAN mirror. There are several other choices under Packages, among them Load package, Select repositories and Install package(s), but the mirror needs to be selected before they are used. The cmprsk package is in the CRAN repository. The user can then install the necessary packages, which will need to be loaded every time a session is started.

B.1.2   Getting help

Under Help in the menu bar one can find PDF manuals as well as information on specific functions. The same information can be found by typing at the prompt:

```
> help (FunctionName)
or
> ?FunctionName
```

For example, for the function that calculates summary statistics, summary, type:

```
> ?summary
```

Almost every function has some examples and these can be seen either in the Help window or by using the function example. For the function mean, type:

```
> example(mean)
mean> x <- c(0:10, 50)
mean> xm <- mean(x)
mean> c(xm, mean(x, trim = 0.1))
[1] 8.75 5.50
mean> data(USArrests)
mean> mean(USArrests, trim = 0.2)

 Murder   Assault   UrbanPop    Rape
   7.42    167.60      66.20   20.16
```

Even though a package is not yet loaded (but is already installed) one can find information on it by typing:

```
> help(package=PackageName)
```

For the package cmprsk the command is:

```
> help(package=cmprsk)
```

B.1.3   Operators in R

The assignment operator in R can be either <- (as shown above) or the usual = sign. Care is needed if one wishes to enquire whether x is less than −1. The sequence

```
> x<-1
```

will be interpreted as an assignment. The correct form is

```
> x<(-1)
```

The assignment operator used in this book is the = sign.

The arithmetic operators are the usual ones: +, -, *, /. The logical operators are: & for 'and', | for 'or', and ! for 'not'. The missing values appear as NAs. An interesting function is is.na, which selects missing values, but is mostly used to select non-missing values. Suppose that x is defined as follows:

```
> x=c(1:4,NA)
> x
[1] 1 2 3 4 NA
> !is.na(x)
[1] TRUE TRUE TRUE TRUE FALSE
> y=x[!is.na(x)]
> y
[1] 1 2 3 4
```

B.1.4   Objects in R

Each object in R is of a specific class. Some examples are: numeric, factor, character, logical, matrix, data frame, list. A number is a vector of length 1:

```
> x=1
> x
[1] 1
```

It can be transformed into a factor by typing

```
> y=as.factor(x)
```

The **class** function can be used to find the type of an object:

```
> class(y)
[1] "factor"
```

x, as defined above, is numeric:

```
> class(x)
[1] "numeric"
```

Some care needs to be exercised when transforming one class into another, since this may give a surprising result. Define an object y of character type:

```
> y=as.character(c(23,12,1,45))
> class(y)
[1] "character"
```

When y is transformed into a numeric object the result is what one would expect:

```
> as.numeric(y)
[1] 23 12  1 45
```

However, if x is defined as a factor:

```
> x=as.factor(c(23,12,1,45))
> class(x)
[1] "factor"
```

its numeric transformation consists of the ranks of its elements:

```
> as.numeric(x)
[1] 3 2 1 4
```

An important feature of R is its ability to work with matrices and vectors. Suppose that x and y are defined as follows:

```
> x=c(1:5)
> x
[1] 1 2 3 4 5
> y=matrix(c(1:20),ncol=4)
> y
```

```
          [,1]    [,2]    [,3]    [,4]
   [1,]      1       6      11      16
   [2,]      2       7      12      17
   [3,]      3       8      13      18
   [4,]      4       9      14      19
   [5,]      5      10      15      20
```

The matrix **y** can be multiplied by 2 by typing

```
> y*2
          [,1]    [,2]    [,3]    [,4]
   [1,]      2      12      22      32
   [2,]      4      14      24      34
   [3,]      6      16      26      36
   [4,]      8      18      28      38
   [5,]     10      20      30      40
```

Matrix-specific operations are also available:

```
> x%*%y
        [,1]    [,2]    [,3]    [,4]
[1,]     55     130     205     280
```

The function `apply` is very helpful when it is desired to calculate a specific quantity by column or row. Applying the `mean` function to **y** gives the average of all 20 values of **y**:

```
> mean(y)
[1] 10.5
```

The `apply` function can be used to calculate the average for each row:

```
> apply(y,1,mean)
[1] 8.5 9.5 10.5 11.5 12.5
```

The sum for each column can be calculated:

```
> apply(y,2,sum)
[1] 15 40 65 90
```

While a matrix has to have all elements of the same class, data frames can accommodate different types of variables. A data frame can be imagined as an ordinary dataset in which the rows are observations and the columns are variables. Thus, some columns could be of class character, some could be factors and some could be numeric. However, the columns need to have the same length. A list is even more general. The elements of a list can have different length and can be of different class.

```
> x=list(c(1:5),c('F','M'),mean(z)<2)
> x
[[1]]
[1] 1 2 3 4 5
[[2]]
[1] "F" "M"
[[3]]
[1] TRUE
> class(x)
[1] "list"
```

All objects created in a session can be listed using

```
> ls()
```

B.1.5   The cmprsk package and datasets

A package, although installed, needs to be loaded every time a new session starts (every time R is invoked). In this book the cmprsk package is used, and it can be loaded either by using the menu bar or by typing:

```
> load(cmprsk)
```

The functions included in the package are listed in Table B.1. To familiarize the reader with this software, a dataset will be read and a data frame created. A way to create a new column in a data frame will also be shown.

In contrast with a package, which has to be loaded for each new session, a dataset needs to be read only once if, when exiting R, the workspace is saved (the user is prompted to do this if desired). If the file containing the dataset tamrt is in C:\datasets\tamrt.txt then one can read it into R by typing:

```
>tamrt=read.table('C:/datasets/tamrt.txt',sep=',',header=T)
```

Note that the assignment operator used is the equal sign (=). The above command creates an object of data.frame class. To see the dataset, type the name, tamrt, at the prompt. To list the variable names one can use the command:

Table B.1   The functions included in `cmprsk` package and their description.

Functions	Description
`cuminc`	Gives estimates of the CIF Performs tests of equality between CIFs (Kalbfleisch and Prentice, 1980; Gray, 1988)
`print.cuminc`	Prints the CIF estimates and their variance obtained with `cnuminc`
`timepoints`	Prints the estimates of the CIF at certain points
`plot.cuminc`	Creates plots for the CIF
`crr`	Performs regression, modeling the hazard of the CIF (Fine and Gray, 1999)
`predict.crr`	Computes the predicted values for the models created with `crr`
`print.crr`	Prints the `crr` output
`plot.predict.crr`	Creates plots for the predicted values obtained in `predict.crr`

```
>names(tamrt)
[1]   "tx"        "pathsize" "hist"     "hgb"     "nodediss" "age"
[7]   "survtime" "stat"     "loctime"  "lcens"   "axltime"  "acens"
[13] "distime"  "dcens"    "maltime"  "mcens"   "hrlevel"  "stnum"
```

A variable in a data.frame can be referred to using $:

```
>tamrt$tx
```

and can be summarized using the command `table` or `summary`:

```
> table(tamrt$tx)
B   T
320 321
> summary(tamrt$age)
   Min.   1st Qu. Median      Mean  3rd Qu.  Max.
  50.00   59.00   67.00     66.45    73.00  88.00
```

The `summary` function can also be applied to the whole data frame to provide summary statistics for each variable:

```
summary(tamrt)
tx        pathsize       hist        hgb         nodediss      age
B:320 Min.   :0.200  DUC :397  Min.   : 96.0  N:106  Min.   :50.00
T:321 1st Qu.:1.000  LOB: 31  1st Qu.:128.0  Y:535  1st Qu.:59.00
```

```
Median :1.500   MED: 5    Median :135.0     Median :67.00
Mean   :1.547   MIX:174   Mean   :135.4     Mean   :66.45
3rd Qu.:2.000   MUC: 16   3rd Qu.:142.0     3rd Qu.:73.00
Max.   :4.500   OTH: 18   Max.   :169.0     Max.   :88.00


      survtime            stat            loctime            lcens
Min.    :0.1615   Min.    :0.00000   Min.    :0.1615   Min.    :0.00000
1st Qu.:4.1697    1st Qu.:0.00000    1st Qu.:3.9973    1st Qu.:0.00000
Median :5.5989    Median :0.00000    Median :5.4100    Median :0.00000
Mean   :5.5260    Mean   :0.07488    Mean   :5.3622    Mean   :0.06084
3rd Qu.:7.0527    3rd Qu.:0.00000    3rd Qu.:6.9405    3rd Qu.:0.00000
Max.   :9.7002    Max.   :1.00000    Max.   :9.7002    Max.   :1.00000


       axltime            acens            distime            dcens
Min.    :0.1561   Min.    :0.00000   Min.    :0.1615   Min.    :0.00000
1st Qu.:4.0794    1st Qu.:0.00000    1st Qu.:4.1205    1st Qu.:0.00000
Median :5.5195    Median :0.00000    Median :5.5414    Median :0.00000
Mean   :5.4670    Mean   :0.02028    Mean   :5.4520    Mean   :0.06396
3rd Qu.:7.0281    3rd Qu.:0.00000    3rd Qu.:7.0226    3rd Qu.:0.00000
Max.   :9.7002    Max.   :1.00000    Max.   :9.7002    Max.   :1.00000


       maltime            mcens            hrlevel            stnum
Min.    :0.1615   Min.    :0.00000   NEG: 46          Min.    : 1
1st Qu.:3.8439    1st Qu.:0.00000    POS:595          1st Qu.:161
Median :5.3525    Median :0.00000                     Median :321
Mean   :5.3062    Mean   :0.09672                     Mean   :321
3rd Qu.:6.8939    3rd Qu.:0.00000                     3rd Qu.:481
Max.   :9.7002    Max.   :1.00000                     Max.   :641
```

Suppose now that it is desired to create a variable in the data frame `tamrt` which represents the time to the first observed event. In the tamoxifen trial the first occurrence of each type of event was recorded. This means, for instance, that if a particular patient had a first local relapse at 2 years, a second local relapse at 2.5 years, and a first distant relapse at 3 years, the second local relapse at 2.5 years would not be recorded. The time to the first event would be the minimum of all times observed. To calculate the minimum of these event times in R, use the `apply` function:

```
>tamrt$dftime=apply(cbind(tamrt$loctime,tamrt$axltime,
tamrt$distime,tamrt$maltime),1,min)
```

The `apply` function has three parameters: a matrix, created here using the command `cbind`, an indicator to specify how to apply the function and the function to be used. The indicator is 1 if the function is applied to the rows or 2 if it is applied to the columns. In this case the minimum for each row is assigned to `tamrt$dftime`.

The work done in a session can be saved in a specific directory. First, the default directory can be changed and then the workspace saved by selecting File from the menu bar and then Save workspace.

The R functions included in Section B.3 are not part of the `cmprsk` package. They can be downloaded from the same website address as the datasets (see Preface) and saved on the local drive. Assuming that, for example, the function `cifDM` is saved in the directory

`C:/rfunctions` under the name `cifDM.txt`, then it can be used after sourcing it in R:

```
> source('c:/rfunctions/cifDM.txt')
```

More details about R software in general can be found in the R manuals and in Fox (2002).

B.2   IMPORTING DATASETS IN SAS

Since SAS is widely used, several SAS macros are included in this book (see Section B.4 and this book's website). To import a dataset which is in the form of a comma delimited text file, the following lines can be run:

```
filename tamrtext 'C:/datasets/tamrt.txt';
proc import out=tamrt datafile=tamrtext dbms=csv replace;
  delimiter=',';getnames=YES;
```

In this way a temporary SAS dataset (`tamrt`) is created using the information from `C:/datasets/tamrt.txt`, which is a comma delimited text file. The names of the variables are on the first line of the file and are imported in the SAS temporary file.

B.3   OTHER PROGRAMS WRITTEN FOR R

B.3.1   CIF variance based on the delta method

```
cifDM=function(time,cens,group=rep(1,length(time)))
{
```

```
# this function calculates the CIF estimates and  #
# their variance based on the delta method        #
```

```
lg=labels(table(group))$group
ng=length(lg)
dd=table(time,cens,group)
tt=sort(unique(time))

for (i in 1:ng)
{

dd1=dd[,,i] ## table of censor, ev, cr
dd2=apply(dd1,1,sum) ## sum for each time point
nrisk=sum(dd2)-cumsum(dd2)
nrisk=c(sum(dd2),nrisk[1:(length(nrisk)-1)])
dev=dd1[,2]
dcr=dd1[,3]
dall=dev+dcr
si=(nrisk-dall)/nrisk
s=cumprod(si)
sminus=c(1,s[1:(length(s)-1)])
fi=dev/nrisk*sminus
f=cumsum(fi)
t1i=dall/(nrisk*(nrisk-dall))
t2i=f*t1i
t3i=f^2*t1i
t4i=sminus^2*(nrisk-dev)*dev/nrisk^3
t5i=sminus*dev/nrisk^2
t6i=f*t5i
t1=cumsum(t1i)
t2=cumsum(t2i)
t3=cumsum(t3i)
t4=cumsum(t4i)
t5=cumsum(t5i)
t6=cumsum(t6i)
v=f^2*t1-2*f*t2+t3+t4-2*f*t5+2*t6

res=data.frame(time=tt,cif=f,var=v,group=rep(lg[i],
  length(v)))
res1=res[dev>0,]
```

```
if (i==1) cifdelta=res1
else cifdelta=list(cifdelta,res1)
}

return(cifdelta)
}
```

B.3.2   Pepe–Mori test for the difference between two CIFs

```
compCIF=function(time,cens,group=rep(1,length(time)))
{
```
```
# this function compares the CIF-s of two groups    #
# it is based on the test presented in the paper     #
# from Statistics in Medicine, 1993, by Pepe and Mori #
```
```
ttau=unlist(by(time,group,max))
tau=min(ttau)
ng=table(group)
lg=labels(ng)$group
dd=table(time,cens,group)
if (dim(dd)[3]!=2) stop("Pepe-Mori test is for two groups")
if (dim(dd)[2]>3) stop("All competing risks should be grouped
under code 2")
if (dim(dd)[2]==2)
{ddd=array(0,dim=c(dim(dd)[1],3,2))
if (sum(cens==0)==0)
{ddd[,2:3,]=dd
        }
if (sum(cens==1)==0)
{warning('There are only competing risks')
ddd[,1,]=dd[,1,]
ddd[,3,]=dd[,2,]
   }
if (sum(cens==2)==0)
{warning('There are no competing risks')
ddd[,1:2,]=dd
        }
    }
if (dim(dd)[2]<2) stop('Either all observations are
  censored or\nthere is only one type of event
  and no censor observations')
dd=ddd
tt=sort(unique(time))
tt1=c(tt[2:length(tt)],NA)
```

```
nt=table(ttl<=tau)[2]
deltat=ttl-tt
dd=dd[1:nt,,]
deltat=deltat[1:nt]
tt=tt[1:nt]

for (i in 1:2)
{

dd1=dd[,,i] ## table of censor, ev, cr
dd2=apply(dd1,1,sum) ## sum for each time point
nrisk=ng[i]-cumsum(c(0,dd2[1:(nt-1)]))
dev=dd1[,2]
dcr=dd1[,3]
dcens=dd1[,1]+dcr
dall=dev+dcr
si=(nrisk-dall)/nrisk
s=cumprod(si)
sminus=c(1,s[1:(length(s)-1)])
fi=dev/nrisk*sminus
f=cumsum(fi)
fcri=dcr/nrisk*sminus
fcr=cumsum(fcri)
Ci=(nrisk-dcens)/nrisk
C=cumprod(Ci)
Cminus=c(1,C[1:(length(C)-1)])

if (i==1)
{nrisk1=nrisk
s1=s
f1=f
fcr1=fcr
C1=C
C1minus=Cminus
dall1=dall
dev1=dev }
if(i==2)
{nrisk2=nrisk
s2=s
f2=f
fcr2=fcr
C2=C
C2minus=Cminus
dall2=dall
dev2=dev}

}
```

```
wi=C1minus*C2minus*sum(ng)/(ng[1]*C1minus+ng[2]*C2minus)
si=wi*(f1-f2)*deltat
s=sqrt(ng[1]*ng[2]/sum(ng))*sum(si)
# for group 1
temp=wi*(1-f1)*deltat
temp[is.na(temp)]=0
t1parti=rev(cumsum(rev(temp)))
temp=wi*f1*deltat
temp[is.na(temp)]=0
t2i=rev(cumsum(rev(temp)))
temp=wi*deltat
temp[is.na(temp)]=0
t3i=fcr1*rev(cumsum(rev(temp)))
t1i=t1parti-t3i
sigma1i=(dev1*t1i^2+(dall1-dev1)*t2i^2)/
  (nrisk1*(nrisk1-1))
sigma1=sum(sigma1i,na.rm=T)

# for group 2
temp=wi*(1-f2)*deltat
temp[is.na(temp)]=0
t1parti=rev(cumsum(rev(temp)))
temp=wi*f2*deltat
temp[is.na(temp)]=0
t2i=rev(cumsum(rev(temp)))
temp=wi*deltat
temp[is.na(temp)]=0
t3i=fcr2*rev(cumsum(rev(temp)))
t1i=t1parti-t3i
sigma2i=(dev2*t1i^2+(dall2-dev2)*t2i^2)/
  (nrisk2*(nrisk2-1))
sigma2=sum(sigma2i,na.rm=T)

sigma=ng[1]*ng[2]*(sigma1+sigma2)/sum(ng)
z=s^2/sigma
pvalue=1-pchisq(z,1)
r=data.frame(chisquare=z,pvalue=pvalue)
row.names(r)=''
return(r)
}
```

B.3.3   Conditional probability and its variance

```
CPvar=function(time,cens,group=rep(1,length(time)))
{
```

```
# this function calculates                          #
#      the CIF for the event of interest            #
#      the CIF for competing risks (fcr)            #
#      the conditional probability                  #
# the variance for the conditional probability      #
#          based on Pepe and Mori-s article in      #
#          Statistics in Medicine, 1993.            #
```

```
lg=labels(table(group))$group
ng=length(lg)
dd=table(time,cens,group)
tt=sort(unique(time))

for (i in 1:ng)
{

dd1=dd[,,i] ## table of censor, ev, cr
dd2=apply(dd1,1,sum) ## sum for each time point
nrisk=sum(dd2)-cumsum(dd2)
nrisk=c(sum(dd2),nrisk[1:(length(nrisk)-1)])
dev=dd1[,2]
dcr=dd1[,3]
dall=dev+dcr
si=(nrisk-dall)/nrisk
s=cumprod(si)
sminus=c(1,s[1:(length(s)-1)])
fi=dev/nrisk*sminus
f=cumsum(fi)
fcri=dcr/nrisk*sminus
fcr=cumsum(fcri)
fcrminus=c(0,fcr[1:(length(fcr)-1)])
cp=f/(1-fcr)

t1i=dev*(1-fcr) 2
t2i=f^ 2*(dall-dev)
v1i=(t1i+t2i)/(nrisk*(nrisk-1))
v1i[nrisk==1]=0
v1=cumsum(v1i)
v=sminus^ 2*v1/((1-fcr)^ 4)

res=data.frame(time=tt,cif=f,fcr,cp,varCP=v,
group=rep(lg[i],length(v)))
res1=res[dall>0,]
if (i==1) cpvar=res1
else cpvar=list(cpvar,res1)
}
return(cpvar)
}
```

B.3.4 Plotting the conditional probability

```
plot.cp=function(aa,xlab='Time to event',
ylab='Conditional probability')
{

## plots the conditional probability #
## aa is an object created with Cpvar  #

ng=length(aa)
m=0

for (i in 1:ng)
{
m=max(m,aa[[i]]$time)
}

for (i in 1:ng)
{
doubletime=sort(c(aa[[i]]$time,aa[[i]]$time))
doublecp=sort(c(aa[[i]]$cp,aa[[i]]$cp))
doubletime=c(0,doubletime)
doublecp=c(0,0,doublecp[1:(length(doublecp)-1)])
if (i==1)
{plot(doubletime,doublecp,xlim=c(0,m),ylim=c(0,1),
xlab=xlab,ylab=ylab,type='l',lty=1)}
else {lines(doubletime,doublecp,lty=i)}
}
}
```

B.3.5 Testing the conditional probability

```
compCP=function(time,cens,group=rep(1,length(time)))
{

# this function compares the CP-s of two groups
# it is based on the test presented in the paper
# from Statistics in Medicine, 1993, by Pepe and Mori

ttau=unlist(by(time,group,max))
tau=min(ttau)
ng=table(group)
lg=labels(ng)$group
dd=table(time,cens,group)
if (dim(dd)[3]!=2) stop('Pepe-Mori test is for two groups')
if (dim(dd)[2]>3) stop('All competing risks should be
grouped under code 2')
```

```
if (dim(dd)$[2]<=2$) stop(''There are either no censored obs
   or \ nno competing risks or no events of interest'')
tt=sort(unique(time))
tt1=c(tt[2:length(tt)],NA)
nt=table(tt1<=tau)[2]
deltat=tt1-tt
dd=dd[1:nt,,]
deltat=deltat[1:nt]
tt=tt[1:nt]

for (i in 1:2)
{

dd1=dd[,,i] ## table of censor, ev, cr
dd2=apply(dd1,1,sum) ## sum for each time point
nrisk=ng[i]-cumsum(c(0,dd2[1:(nt-1)]))
dev=dd1[,2]
dcr=dd1[,3]
dcens=dd1[,1]+dcr
dall=dev+dcr
si=(nrisk-dall)/nrisk
s=cumprod(si)
sminus=c(1,s[1:(length(s)-1)])
fi=dev/nrisk*sminus
f=cumsum(fi)
fcri=dcr/nrisk*sminus
fcr=cumsum(fcri)
cp=f/(1-fcr)
Ci=(nrisk-dcens)/nrisk
C=cumprod(Ci)
Cminus=c(1,C[1:(length(C)-1)])

if (i==1)
{nrisk1=nrisk
s1=s
f1=f
fcr1=fcr
C1=C
CP1=cp
C1minus=Cminus
dall1=dall
dev1=dev}
if (i==2)
{nrisk2=nrisk
s2=s
f2=f
```

```
fcr2=fcr
C2=C
CP2=cp
C2minus=Cminus
dall2=dall
dev2=dev}

}

wi=C1minus*C2minus*sum(ng)/(ng[1]*C1minus+ng[2]*C2minus)
si=wi*(CP1-CP2)*deltat
s=sqrt(ng[1]*ng[2]/sum(ng))*sum(si)

# for group 1
temp=wi*s1*deltat/(1-fcr1)**2
temp[is.na(temp)]=0
tparti=rev(cumsum(rev(temp)))

sigma1i=tparti**2*(dev1*(1-fcr1)**2+(dall1-
dev1)*f1**2)/(nrisk1*(nrisk1-1))
sigma1=sum(sigma1i,na.rm=T)
# for group 2
temp=wi*s2*deltat/(1-fcr2)**2
temp[is.na(temp)]=0
tparti=rev(cumsum(rev(temp)))

sigma2i=tparti**2*(dev2*(1-fcr2)**2+(dall2-
dev2)*f2**2)/(nrisk2*(nrisk2-1))
sigma2=sum(sigma2i,na.rm=T)
sigma=ng[1]*ng[2]*(sigma1+sigma2)/sum(ng)
z=sn^ 2/sigma
pvalue=1-pchisq(z,1)
r=data.frame(chisquare=z,pvalue=pvalue)
row.names(r)=''
return(r)
}
```

B.3.6 Calculating the conditional probability of observing the event of interest in a time period knowing that the patient was free of any event at the beginning of the period

```
btvarCP2=function(time,cens,t1,t2,nbt,s0=0,alpha=0.05)
{
```

```
# bootstrap time and cens to obtain       #
# an estimate of the variance             #
```

```
# and the confidence intervals for the     #
# probability to fail beetween t1 and t2    #
#     from the event coded as 1 in cens     #
#     knowing that the patient is free      #
#     of any event at time t1               #
```
```
# time=time to first failure                #
# cens=1 for event of interest              #
#       2 for competing risk                #
#       0 for no event                      #
# t1 and t2 the time window for which       #
#    the conditional probability is calculated#
# nbt=number of bootstrap repetitions       #
# s0=the seed (for exact replication)       #
```
```
n=length(time)
bt=function()
  {
idx=sample(c(1:n),size=n,replace=T)
tbt=time[idx]
cbt=cens[idx]
fitbt=cuminc(tbt,cbt)
sumbt=timepoints(fitbt,times=c(t1,t2))
cp2=(sumbt$est[1,2]-sumbt$est[1,1])/(1-sumbt$est[2,1]-
sumbt$est[1,1])
return(cp2)
  }
CP2=vector('numeric',nbt)
set.seed(s0)
for (i in 1:nbt) CP2[i]=bt()
varCP2=var(CP2)
fit=cuminc(time,cens)
sumfit=timepoints(fit,times=c(t1,t2))
cpw=(sumfit$est[1,2]-sumfit$est[1,1])/(1-sumfit$est[2,1]-
sumfit$est[1,1])
z=qnorm(1-alpha/2)
A=z*sqrt(varCP2)/(cpw*log(cpw))
loA=exp(-A)
upA=exp(A)
lo=cpw^loA
up=cpw^upA
r=data.frame(CPw=cpw,varCPw=varCP2,'L95%CI'=lo,'U95%
CI'=up)
row.names(r)=''
return(r)
}
```

B.3.7   Comparing two types of risk in the same population

```
kly=function(time,cens)
{
```

```
# based on Kochar, Lam and Yip      #
# Lifetime Data Analysis, 2002       #
```

```
# time=time to first event            #
# cens=censor variable                #
#        1=one type of event          #
#        2=another type of event      #
#        0=the rest of events and     #
#        censored records             #
################################ ####

dd0=table(time,cens)
if (sum(cens==0)==0) {dd=cbind(rep(0,nrow(dd0)),dd0)}
else {dd=dd0}
if (sum(cens==1)==0 | sum(cens==2)==0 | sum(cens>2)>0)
{stop ('Codes for events should be 1 or 2')}
n=length(time)
sigma=sqrt(n*sum(cens>0))
nt=apply(dd,1,sum)
ntt=cumsum(nt)
atrisk=n-ntt
lnti=(dd[,3]-dd[,2])
lnt=cumsum(lnti)
k=nrow(dd)
maxlnt=vector('numeric',k)

for (i in 1:k)
{
maxlnt[i]=max(abs(lnt-lnt[i]))
}

cnw=sqrt(n)*max(maxlnt)/sigma
## for C, (without absolute value)
pcnw=function(c)
{
k=c(0:15)
parti=(-1)^k*exp(-pi^ 2*(2*k+1) 2/(8*cc^ 2))/(2*k+1)
p=sum(parti)*4/pi
return(p)
}
```

```
## for Cstar (with absolute value)
ph=function(z)
{
f1=function(x1,x2,k,xi)
{
ki=c(1:k)
x=c((x1*xi):(x2*xi))/xi
n=length(x)
h=vector('numeric',n)

for (i in 1:n)
{
h[i]=sum(8*(-1)^(ki-1)*ki^2*dnorm(ki*x[i]))
}

parth=sum(h)/xi
return(parth)}

if (z<=0.1)
ph=f1(0.01,z,1000,100)
else if (z<=0.5)
ph=f1(0.01,0.1,1000,100)+f1(0.11,z,100,100)
else ph=f1(0.01,0.1,1000,100)+f1(0.11,0.5,100,100)+
f1(0.51,z,30,1000)
return(ph)
}

pvalue=1-ph(cnw)
if (pvalue>=0.00001) r=data.frame(cnw,pvalue)
if (pvalue<0.00001) r=data.frame(cnw,pvalue='p-value<0.00001')
row.names(r)=''
return(r)
 }
```

B.3.8   Calculating the power

```
power=function(N,a,f,pi,theta=NA,t0,type='CSH',alpha=0.05,
KMev0=NA,KMcr0=NA,KMev1=NA,KMcr1=NA,
CIFev0=NA,CIFcr0=NA,CIFev1=NA,CIFcr1=NA)
{
#### CALCULATES POWER
## for difference between two groups
## need to import the function eqsolve
```

```
## n=total number of patients which will be accrued
## theta=hazard ratio:
```

```
##   if type=CSH then is the ratio of the cause specific hazrard
##   if type=HCIF then is the ratio of the hazards of CIF
## a=accrual time,
## f=follow-up time,
## t0=time at which KM and CIF are given
## a,f and t0 are all in the same units
## CIFev0=CIF for event in standard group at t0
## CIFcr0=CIF for competing risks in standard group at t0
## CIFev1=CIF for event in experimental group at t0
## CIFcr1=CIF for competing risks in experimental group at t0
## KMev0=KM estimate for free of event in standard group at t0
## KMcr0=KM estimate for free of event in standard group at t0
## KMev1=KM estimate for free of event in experimental group
at t0
## KMcr1=KM estimate for free of event in experimental group
at t0
## pi=proportion in standard group, default=0.5
## alpha= alpha level, default=0.05
```

```
##### ASSUMPTIONS #####
## exponential distribution for both groups and both events
## independence between the types of events
## the competing risks the same in the standard and competing
risks
```

```
if (!is.na(KMev0) & !is.na(KMcr0))
   {
lev0=-log(KMev0)/t0
lcr0=-log(KMcr0)/t0
   }
if (is.na(KMev0) & is.na(KMcr0) & !is.na(CIFev0) &
!is.na(CIFcr0))
   {
CIF0=CIFev0+CIFcr0
part=-log(1-CIF0)/(t0*CIF0)
lev0=CIFev0*part
lcr0=CIFcr0*part
   }

if (is.na(lev0) | is.na(lcr0)) stop('Not enough information
given')
lev1=NA
lcr1=lcr0

if (!is.na(KMev1) & !is.na(KMcr1))
   {
lev1=-log(KMev1)/t0
```

```
lcr1=-log(KMcr1)/t0
  }

if (is.na(KMev1) & is.na(KMcr1) & !is.na(CIFev1) &
!is.na(CIFcr1))
  {
CIF1=CIFev1+CIFcr1
part=-log(1-CIF1)/(t0*CIF1)
lev1=CIFev1*part
lcr1=CIFcr1*part
  }

if (is.na(lev1) & is.na(theta)) stop('theta is missing')
if (type=='CSH' & !is.na(theta)) lev1=lev0/theta
if (type=='HCIF' & !is.na(theta)) CIFev1=1-(1-CIFev0)**(1/theta)
if (is.na(lev1)) lev1=eqsolve(CIFev1,lcr1,t0)
l0=lev0+lcr0
l1=lev1+lcr1

if (is.na(theta) & type=='CSH') theta=lev0/lev1
if (is.na(CIFev0)) CIFev0=lev0/l0*(1-exp(-l0*t0))
if (is.na(CIFev1)) CIFev1=lev1/l1*(1-exp(-l1*t0))
if (is.na(theta) & type=='HCIF') theta=log(1-CIFev0)/
  log(1-CIFev1)
pev0=lev0/l0*(1-(exp(-l0*f)-exp(-l0*(a+f)))/(l0*a))
pev1=lev1/l1*(1-(exp(-l1*f)-exp(-l1*(a+f)))/(l1*a))
pev=pev0*pi+pev1*(1-pi)
nev=N*pev

zalpha=qnorm(1-alpha/2)
zbeta=sqrt(nev*pi*(1-pi))*abs(log(theta))-zalpha
power=pnorm(zbeta)
return(power)
}

eqsolve=function(fev,lcr,t0)
{
lev1=0.0001
lev2=2
k=0
f1=fev-lev1/(lcr+lev1)*(1-exp(-(lcr+lev1)*t0))
f2=fev-lev2/(lcr+lev2)*(1-exp(-(lcr+lev2)*t0))
if (f1*f2>0) stop('Either lambda is much too high or CIF is
much too small')
fm=10
while (abs(fm)>0.000001)
  {
if (k>10000)
  {
```

```
stop('No convergence')
  }
levm=lev1+(lev2-lev1)/2
fm=fev-levm/(lcr+levm)*(1-exp(-(lcr+levm)*t0))
if (f1*fm<0)
  {
lev2=levm
f2=fm
k=k+1
  }
if (f2*fm<0)
  {
lev1=levm
f1=fm
k=k+1
      }
  }

r=round(levm,4)
return(r)
}
```

B.4   SAS MACROS FOR COMPETING RISK ANALYSIS

B.4.1   Cumulative incidence and conditional probability

```
%macro cuminc(ds= , time= , cenvble= ,interest=, group=) ;
```

```
this macro calculates:
      the CIF for the event of interest
      the variance for CIF based on the delta method
      the conditional probability (CP)
      the variance for conditional probability based
          on Pepe & Mori, stat in med, 1993
this macro creates the graph for
      the CIF for event of interest
      and calculates the conditional probability.
```

```
macro parameters:

1. ds
the name of the input dataset.
```

2. time
the name of the time variable

3. cenvble.
the name of the variable with the censoring/event codes
in order to use this macro, censored observations must
be coded as 0 (zero) and events must have numeric
codes,although they need not be consecutive.

4. interest
denotes the value of the censoring variable (cenvble)
that is of primary interest.the macro produces printed
results including a listing of the cif for each group
and a graph of the cif for the event of interest
for each group. it does not calculate or produce
output for the events other than the one of interest.

5. group
represents the grouping variable.
the group codes can be either character or numeric.

the variance of CIF is calcualted based on
the delta method
the variance of CP is calculated based on
    the formula given in the Pepe and Mori 1993 paper

```
title ' ' ;
footnote ' ' ;

proc sort data = &ds (keep = &time &cenvble &group)
out = sorted ;
by &group &time ;
run ;

data sorted summary ;
set sorted end = eof ;
by &group &time ;
retain grpcat 0 grpn freq totevt totcen totint tototh ;
   add1 = first.&group ;
    grpcat + add1 ;
if eof then call symput ('grpcat',grpcat) ;
if first.&group then grpn = 1 ;
else grpn = grpn+1 ;
if last.&group then call symput ('grpn'||
trim(put(grpcat,1.)), grpn ) ;
if &cenvble = 0 then cenxyz = 0 ;
else if &cenvble = &interest then cenxyz = 1 ;
```

```
else if &cenvble not in (0, &interest) then cenxyz = 2 ;
if first.&time then do ;
freq = 1 ;
totint = (cenxyz = 1) ;
tototh = (cenxyz = 2) ;
end ;
else do ;
freq = freq + 1 ;
totint = totint + (cenxyz = 1) ;
tototh = tototh + (cenxyz = 2) ;
end ;
totevt = totint + tototh ;
output sorted ;
if last.&time then output summary ;
drop add1 grpn ;
run ;
data summary1;
set summary ;
by &group &time ;
if first.&group then do i = 1 to 1 ;
output ;
end ;
output ;
run ;
data summary2 ;
set summary1 ;
by &group ;
retain surv atrisk sprev cif f2 t2 p4 p5 p1 p2 p3 v;
if i = 1 then do ;
&time=0 ; &cenvble=. ;
freq=0 ; totevt=0 ;
totint=0 ; tototh = 0 ;
end ;
if first.&group then do ;
atrisk = input(compress(trim(symget('grpn'||
trim(put(grpcat,1.)))))),8.);
sprev = 1 ;
surv = 1-totevt/atrisk ;
cif = totint / atrisk ;
f2 = tototh / atrisk ;
t2 = (totint/atrisk**2)*(1-totint/atrisk) ;
p1 = totevt/(atrisk*(atrisk-totevt)) ;
p2 = cif*totevt/(atrisk*(atrisk-totevt)) ;
p3 = (cif**2)*totevt/(atrisk*(atrisk-totevt)) ;
p4 = totint/(atrisk**2) ;
p5 = (cif*totint)/(atrisk**2) ;
```

```
v = (totint*(1-f2)**2+tototh*cif**2)/(atrisk*(atrisk-1));
atrisk = atrisk - freq ;
end ;
else do ;
sprev = surv ;
surv = surv*(1-totevt/atrisk) ;
cif = cif + sprev*(totint/atrisk) ;
f2 = f2 + sprev*(tototh/atrisk) ;
t2 = t2 + (sprev**2)*(totint/atrisk**2)*(1-totint/atrisk) ;
p1 = p1 + totevt/(atrisk*(atrisk-totevt)) ;
p2 = p2 + cif*totevt/(atrisk*(atrisk-totevt)) ;
p3 = p3 + (cif**2)*totevt/(atrisk*(atrisk-totevt)) ;
p4 = p4 + sprev*totint/(atrisk**2) ;
p5 = p5 + (sprev*cif*totint)/(atrisk**2) ;
if atrisk>1 then
v=v+(totint*(1-f2)**2+tototh*cif**2)/(atrisk*(atrisk-1));
else v=v;
atrisk = atrisk - freq ;
end ;
drop &cenvble cenxyz i grpcat ;
run ;
data summary3 ;
set summary2 ;
vardelta = (cif**2)*p1 - 2*cif*p2 + p3 + t2 -2*cif*p4 + 2*p5 ;
cp = cif /(1-f2) ;
varcp = (sprev**2/(1-f2)**4)*v;
run ;
proc report data = summary3 nowd colwidth=12
spacing = 2 headline headskip split='*' ;
column &time atrisk totint totevt cif vardelta cp varcp;
define cif / display 'CIF for*type &interest *events'
format=8.6 ;
define vardelta / display 'Variance*for CIF*type &interest
*events'
format=8.6;
define totint /display 'Number*of*type &interest*events'
format=6. ;
define totevt / display 'Total*number*of events' format=7. ;
define atrisk / display 'Number*left' format=6. ;
define cp / display 'CP for*type &interest *events'
format=8.6 ;
define varcp / display 'Variance*for CP*type &interest
*events' format=8.6 ;
by &group ;
where totevt>0;
run ;
```

```
symbol1   c=default   i=stepslj   l=1   w=2   v=none ;
symbol2   c=default   i=stepslj   l=2   w=2   v=none ;
symbol3   c=default   i=stepslj   l=3   w=2   v=none ;
symbol4   c=default   i=stepslj   l=4   w=2   v=none ;
symbol5   c=default   i=stepslj   l=5   w=2   v=none ;
symbol6   c=default   i=stepslj   l=6   w=2   v=none ;
symbol7   c=default   i=stepslj   l=7   w=2   v=none ;
axis2 color=black
label=('CIF' font=swissl h=1 c=black)
width=2.0
value=(font=swissl)
style=1 ;
legend1 position=(top left inside)
down = &grpcat
label=(font=swissl h=0.7 c=black)
value=(font=swissl h=0.7 c=black)
mode=protect ;

proc gplot data = summary3 ;
plot cif * &time =&group /
haxis = axis1 vaxis = axis2 frame
legend = legend1 ;
title h=1.5 c=black f=swissl ''CIF for event &&interest by
&&group'' ;
run ;
axis2 color=black
label=('cp' font=swissl h=1 c=black)
width=2.0
value=(font=swissl)
style=1 ;
proc gplot data = summary3 ;
plot cp * &time =&group /
haxis = axis1 vaxis = axis2 frame
legend = legend1 ;
title h=1.5 c=black f=swissl 'CP for event &&interest by
&&group' ;
run ;
%mend ;
```

B.4.2   Pepe–Mori test for the comparison of two CIFs

```
%macro compcif(ds=, time=, cens=, group=,val1=,val2=);
```

```
It compares the CIF between two groups
It is based on the test described in
Pepe and Mori paper Statistics in Medicine 1993
```

```
ds=data set
time= time to first event observed
cens= censor variable coded as:
          1= event of interest
          2= competing risks type of event
          0= censored (no failure observed)
group=group variable coded as val1 and val2
```

```
data d1;set &ds;
if &cens in (0,2) then c02=1;else c02=0;
if &cens ^ in (0,1) then dcr=1;else dcr=0;
if &cens=1 then dev=1;else dev=0;


data dg1;set d1;if &group=&val1;keep &time c02 dev dcr;
proc means data=dg1 sum noprint;
var c02 dev dcr ;class &time;
output out=dg11 sum=c021 dev1 dcr1 ;
data dg11;set dg11;if _type_=1;keep &time c021 dev1 dcr1;


data dg2;set d1;if &group=&val2; keep &time c02 dev dcr;
proc means data=dg2 sum noprint;
var c02 dev dcr ;class &time;
output out=dg21 sum=c022 dev2 dcr2 ;
data dg21;set dg21;if _type_=1;keep &time c022 dev2 dcr2;


proc means data=d1 noprint;var &time;class &group;
output out=d2 max=tau;
data d21;set d2;if &group=&val1;rename _freq_=n1
tau=tau1;keep freq tau;
data d22;set d2;if &group=&val2;rename _freq_=n2
tau=tau2;keep freq tau;
data d2;merge d21 d22;tau=min(tau1,tau2);keep n1 n2 tau;
data dg;merge dg11 dg21;by &time;
data dg;set dg;
if dev1=. then dev1=0;if dcr1=. then dcr1=0;if c021=. then
c021=0;
if dev2=. then dev2=0;if dcr2=. then dcr2=0;if c022=. then
c022=0;
data dg;set dg;if _n_=1 then set d2;if &time<=tau;
data dg;set dg;retain atrisk1 s1 c1 f1 fcr1 atrisk2 s2 c2
f2 fcr2;
c021m=lag(c021);dev1m=lag(dev1);c022m=lag(c022);
 dev2m=lag(dev2);
```

```
if _n_=1 then do;
atrisk1=n1;
s1=(atrisk1-dev1-dcr1)/atrisk1;
c1=(atrisk1-c021)/atrisk1;
f1=dev1/atrisk1;
fcr1=dcr1/atrisk1;
atrisk2=n2;
s2=(atrisk2-dev2-dcr2)/atrisk2;
c2=(atrisk2-c022)/atrisk2;
f2=dev2/atrisk2;
fcr2=dcr2/atrisk2;
end;
else do;
atrisk1=atrisk1-c021m-dev1m;
s1=s1*(atrisk1-dev1-dcr1)/atrisk1;
c1=c1*(atrisk1-c021)/atrisk1;
atrisk2=atrisk2-c022m-dev2m;
s2=s2*(atrisk2-dev2-dcr2)/atrisk2;
c2=c2*(atrisk2-c022)/atrisk2;
end;
s1m=lag(s1);s2m=lag(s2); c1m=lag(c1);c2m=lag(c2);
if _n_=1 then do;
s1m=1;s2m=1; c1m=1;c2m=1;
end;

if _n_>1 then do;
f1=f1+dev1/atrisk1*s1m;
fcr1=fcr1+dcr1/atrisk1*s1m;
f2=f2+dev2/atrisk2*s2m;
fcr2=fcr2+dcr2/atrisk2*s2m;
end;

w=c1m*c2m*(n1+n2)/(n1*c1m+n2*c2m);
data temp;set dg;keep &time;
proc sort data=temp;by descending &time ;
data temp;set temp;timem=lag(&time);
proc sort data=temp;by &time ;
data dg;merge temp dg;by &time;

data dg;set dg;
retain v1part v21part v22part;
if timem=. then delete;
deltat=timem-&time;
spart=w*(f1-f2)*deltat;

** variance;
if _n_=1 then do;
```

```
v1i=w*deltat;
v21i=v1i*f1;
v22i=v1i*f2;
v1part=w*deltat;
v21part=v1i*f1;
v22part=v1i*f2;
end;
else do;
v1i=w*deltat;
v21i=v1i*f1;
v22i=v1i*f2;
v1part=v1part+w*deltat;
v21part=v21part+v1i*f1;
v22part=v22part+v1i*f2;
end;

data dlast;set dg end=last;if last;
keep v1part v21part v22part;rename v1part=v1tot
v21part=v21tot v22part=v22tot;
data dg;set dg;if _n_=1 then set dlast;
data dg;set dg;
v1=v1tot-v1part+v1i;
v21=v21tot-v21part+v21i;
v22=v22tot-v22part+v22i;
v11=(1-fcr1)*v1-v21;
v12=(1-fcr2)*v1-v22;
sigma1=(v11**2*dev1+v21**2*dcr1)/(atrisk1*(atrisk1-1));
sigma2=(v12**2*dev2+v22**2*dcr2)/(atrisk2*(atrisk2-1));
proc means data=dg noprint;var spart sigma1 sigma2;
output out=var sum=s sigma1 sigma2;
data var;set var;keep s sigma1 sigma2;

data result;merge var d2;
s=s*sqrt(n1*n2/(n1+n2));
sigma=n1*n2/(n1+n2)*(sigma1+sigma2);
chisq=s**2/sigma;
pvalue=1-probchi(chisq,1);

proc report data=dg nowd colwidth=12 spacing=2 headline
headskip split='*';
column &time atrisk1 dev1 dcr1 f1 fcr1 ;
define &time/display 'Time' format=7.2;
define atrisk1/display 'Number*at risk' format=7.;
define dev1/display 'Number*events of*interest'
format=9.;
define dcr1/display 'Number*competing*risks' format=9.;
```

```
define f1/display ''CIF*event of*interest'' format=8.6;
define fcr1/display ''CIF*competing*risk'' format=9.6;
title1 ''Estimates for group &val1'';
run;

proc report data=dg nowd colwidth=12 spacing=2 headline
headskip split='*';
column &time atrisk2 dev2 dcr2 f2 fcr2 ;
define &time/display 'Time' format=7.2;
define atrisk2/display 'Number*at risk' format=7.;
define dev2/display 'Number*events of*interest' format=9.;
define dcr2/display 'Number*competing*risks' format=9.;
define f2/display 'CIF*event of*interest' format=8.6;
define fcr2/display 'CIF*competing*risk' format=9.6;
title1 'Estimates for group &val2';
run;

proc report data=result nowd colwidth=12 spacing=2 headline
headskip split='*';
column n1 n2 s chisq pvalue;
define n1/display 'N*Group*&val1' format=7.;
define n2/display 'N*Group*&val2' format=7.;
define s/display 'Score' format=13.4;
define chisq/display 'Chi-square' format=13.4;
define pvalue/display 'p-value' format=7.5;
%mend;
```

B.4.3   Pepe–Mori test for the comparison of two CPs

```
%macro compcp(ds=, time=, cens=, group=, val1=, val2=,);
```

```
It compares the CP between two groups
It is based on the test described in
Pepe and Mori paper Statistics in Medicine 1993
```

```
ds=data set
time= time to first event observed
cens= censor variable coded as:
           1= event of interest
           2= competing risks type of event
           0= censored (no failure observed)
group=group variable coded as val1 and val2
```

```
data d1;set &ds;
if &cens in (0,2) then c02=1;else c02=0;
if &cens ^ in (0,1) then dcr=1;else dcr=0;
if &cens=1 then dev=1;else dev=0;
```

```
data dg1;set d1;if &group=&val1;keep &time c02 dev dcr;
proc means data=dg1 sum noprint;
var c02 dev dcr ;class &time;
output out=dg11 sum=c021 dev1 dcr1 ;
data dg11;set dg11;if _type_=1;keep &time c021 dev1 dcr1;


data dg2;set d1;if &group=&val2; keep &time c02 dev dcr;
proc means data=dg2 sum noprint;
var c02 dev dcr ;class &time;
output out=dg21 sum=c022 dev2 dcr2 ;
data dg21;set dg21;if _type_=1;keep &time c022 dev2 dcr2;


proc means data=d1 noprint;var &time;class &group;
output out=d2 max=tau;
data d21;set d2;if &group=&val1;rename _freq_=n1
tau=tau1;keep freq tau;
data d22;set d2;if &group=&val2;rename _freq_=n2
tau=tau2;keep freq tau;
data d2;merge d21 d22;tau=min(tau1,tau2);keep n1 n2 tau;
data dg;merge dg11 dg21;by &time;
data dg;set dg;
if dev1=. then dev1=0;if dcr1=. then dcr1=0;if c021=. then
c021=0;
if dev2=. then dev2=0;if dcr2=. then dcr2=0;if c022=. then
c022=0;
data dg;set dg;if _n_=1 then set d2;if &time<=tau;
data dg;set dg;retain atrisk1 s1 c1 f1 fcr1 atrisk2 s2 c2
f2 fcr2;
c021m=lag(c021);dev1m=lag(dev1);c022m=lag(c022);
 dev2m=lag(dev2);
if _n_=1 then do;
atrisk1=n1;
s1=(atrisk1-dev1-dcr1)/atrisk1;
c1=(atrisk1-c021)/atrisk1;
f1=dev1/atrisk1;
fcr1=dcr1/atrisk1;
cp1=f1/(1-fcr1);
atrisk2=n2;
s2=(atrisk2-dev2-dcr2)/atrisk2;
c2=(atrisk2-c022)/atrisk2;
f2=dev2/atrisk2;
fcr2=dcr2/atrisk2;
cp2=f2/(1-fcr2);
end;
```

```
else do;
atrisk1=atrisk1-c021m-dev1m;
s1=s1*(atrisk1-dev1-dcr1)/atrisk1;
c1=c1*(atrisk1-c021)/atrisk1;
atrisk2=atrisk2-c022m-dev2m;
s2=s2*(atrisk2-dev2-dcr2)/atrisk2;
c2=c2*(atrisk2-c022)/atrisk2;
end;
s1m=lag(s1);s2m=lag(s2); c1m=lag(c1);c2m=lag(c2);
if _n_=1 then do;
s1m=1;s2m=1; c1m=1;c2m=1;
end;

if _n_>1 then do;
f1=f1+dev1/atrisk1*s1m;
fcr1=fcr1+dcr1/atrisk1*s1m;
cp1=f1/(1-fcr1);
f2=f2+dev2/atrisk2*s2m;
fcr2=fcr2+dcr2/atrisk2*s2m;
cp2=f2/(1-fcr2);
end;

w=c1m*c2m*(n1+n2)/(n1*c1m+n2*c2m);
data temp;set dg;keep &time;
proc sort data=temp;by descending &time ;
data temp;set temp;timem=lag(&time);
proc sort data=temp;by &time ;
data dg;merge temp dg;by &time;
data dg;set dg;
retain v1part v2part ;
if timem=. then delete;
deltat=timem-&time;
spart=w*(cp1-cp2)*deltat;

v1i=(s1*w*deltat)/(1-fcr1)**2;
v2i=(s2*w*deltat)/(1-fcr2)**2;

** variance;
if _n_=1 then do;
v1part=v1i;
v2part=v2i;
end;
else do;
v1part=v1part+v1i;
v2part=v2part+v2i;
end;
```

```
data dlast;set dg end=last;if last;
keep v1part v2part;rename v1part=v1tot v2part=v2tot ;
data dg;set dg;if _n_=1 then set dlast;
data dg;set dg;
v1=v1tot-v1part+v1i;
v2=v2tot-v2part+v2i;
sigma1=(v1**2)*((1-fcr1)**2*dev1+f1**2*dcr1)/
(atrisk1*(atrisk1-1));
sigma2=(v2**2)*((1-fcr2)**2*dev2+f2**2*dcr2)/
(atrisk2*(atrisk2-1));
proc means data=dg noprint;var spart sigma1 sigma2;
output out=var sum=s sigma1 sigma2;
data var;set var;keep s sigma1 sigma2;

data result;merge var d2;
s=s*sqrt(n1*n2/(n1+n2));
sigma=n1*n2/(n1+n2)*(sigma1+sigma2);
chisq=s**2/sigma;
pvalue=1-probchi(chisq,1);

proc report data=dg nowd colwidth=12 spacing=2 headline
headskip split='*';
column &time atrisk1 dev1 dcr1 f1 fcr1 cp1 ;
define &time/display ''Time'' format=7.2;
define atrisk1/display ''Number*at risk'' format=7.;
define dev1/display ''Number*events of*interest'' format=9.;
define dcr1/display ''Number*competing*risks'' format=9.;
define f1/display ''CIF*event of*interest'' format=9.6;
define fcr1/display ''CIF*competing*risk'' format=9.6;
define cp1/display ''Conditional*probability'' format=11.6;
title1 ''Estimates for group &val1'';
run;

proc report data=dg nowd colwidth=12 spacing=2 headline
headskip split='*';
column &time atrisk2 dev2 dcr2 f2 fcr2 cp2;
define &time/display 'Time' format=7.2;
define atrisk2/display 'Number*at risk' format=7.;
define dev2/display 'Number*events of*interest' format=9.;
define dcr2/display 'Number*competing*risks' format=9.;
define f2/display 'CIF*event of*interest' format=9.6;
define fcr2/display 'CIF*competing*risk' format=9.6;
define cp2/display 'Conditional*probability' format=11.6;
title1 'Estimates for group &val2';
run;
```

```
proc report data=result nowd colwidth=12 spacing=2 headline
headskip split='*';
column n1 n2 s chisq pvalue;
define n1/display 'N*Group*&val1' format=7.;
define n2/display 'N*Group*&val2' format=7.;
define s/display 'Score' format=13.4;
define chisq/display 'Chi-square' format=13.4;
define pvalue/display 'p-value' format=7.5;
title1 'Comparison of the conditional probabilities';
run;

%mend;
```

Statistics in Practice

Human and Biological Sciences

Berger – Selection Bias and Covariate Imbalance in Randomized Clinical Trials
Brown and Prescott – Applied Mixed Models in Medicine
Chevret (Ed) – Statistical Methods for Dose-Finding Experiments
Ellenberg, Fleming and DeMets – Data Monitoring Committees in Clinical Trials: A Practical Perspective
Lawson, Browne and Vidal Rodeiro – Disease Mapping with WinBUGS and MLwiN
Lui – Statistical Estimation of Epidemiological Risk
*Marubini and Valsecchi – Analysing Survival Data from Clinical Trials and Observation Studies
O'Hagan – Uncertain Judgements: Eliciting Experts' Probabilities
Parmigiani – Modeling in Medical Decision Making: A Bayesian Approach
Pintilie – Competing Risks: A Practical Perspective
Senn – Cross-over Trials in Clinical Research, Second Edition
Senn – Statistical Issues in Drug Development
Spiegelhalter, Abrams and Myles – Bayesian Approaches to Clinical Trials and Health-Care Evaluation
Whitehead – Design and Analysis of Sequential Clinical Trials, Revised Second Edition
Whitehead – Meta-Analysis of Controlled Clinical Trials
Willan – Statistical Analysis of Cost-effectiveness Data

Earth and Environmental Sciences

Buck, Cavanagh and Litton – Bayesian Approach to Interpreting Archaeological Data
Glasbey and Horgan – Image Analysis in the Biological Sciences
Helsel – Nondetects and Data Analysis: Statistics for Censored Environmental Data
McBride – Using Statistical Methods for Water Quality Management
Webster and Oliver – Geostatistics for Environmental Scientists

Industry, Commerce and Finance

Aitken and Taroni – Statistics and the Evaluation of Evidence for Forensic Scientists, Second Edition
Balding – Weight-of-evidence for Forensic DNA Profiles
Lehtonen and Pahkinen – Practical Methods for Design and Analysis of Complex Surveys, Second Edition
Ohser and Mücklich – Statistical Analysis of Microstructures in Materials Science
Taroni, Aitken, Garbolino and Biedermann – Bayesian Networks and Probabilistic Inference in Forensic Science

*Now available in paperback

References

Aalen, O. (1978a). Nonparametric estimation of partial transition probabilities in multiple decrement models. *Annals of Statistics*, **6**, 534–545.

Aalen, O. (1978b). Nonparametric inference for a family of counting processes. *Annals of Statistics*, **6**, 701–726.

Allison, P. (1995) *Survival Analysis Using the SAS System: A Practical Guide*. Cary, NC: BBU Press, SAS Institute.

Benichou, J. and Gail, M. H. (1990). Estimates of absolute cause-specific risk in cohort studies. *Biometrics*, **46**, 813–826.

Bernoulli, D. (1760). Essai d'une nouvelle analyse de la mortalité causée par la petite vérole, et des avantages de l'inoculation pour la prévenir. *Mémoir de l'Academie Royale de Science*. 1–45.

Breslow, N. (1974). Covariance analysis of censored survival data. *Biometrics*, **30**, 89–99.

Cantor, A. (2003) *SAS Survival Analysis Techniques for Medical Research*. Cary, NC: BBU Press, SAS Institute.

Caplan, R. J., Pajak, T. F. and Cox, J. D. (1994). Analysis of probability and risk of cause-specific failure. *International Journal of Radiation Oncology, Biology, Phystcs*, **29**, 1183–1186.

Choudhury, J. B. (2002). Non-parametric confidence interval estimation for competing risks analysis: application to contraceptive data. *Statistics in Medicine*, **21**, 1129–1144.

Collett, D. (2003) *Modelling Survival Data in Medical Research*. Boca Raton, FL: Chapman & Hall/CRC.

Couban, S., Simpson, D. R., Barnett, M. J., Bredeson, C., Hubesch, L., Kang, H. L., Shore, T. B., Walker, I. R., Browett, P., Messner, H. A., Panzarella, T. and Lipton, J. H. (2002). A randomized multicenter comparison of bone marrow and peripheral blood in recipients of

Competing Risks: A Practical Perspective   M. Pintilie
© 2006 John Wiley & Sons, Ltd

matched sibling allogeneic transplants for myeloid malignancies. *Blood*, **100**, 1525–531.

Cox, D. R. (1972). Regression models and life-tables. *Journal of the Royal Statistical Society, Series B*, **34**, 187–220.

Cox, D. R. and Oakes, D. (1984) *Analysis of Survival Data*. London: Chapman & Hall.

Crowder, M. (1996). Some tests based on extreme values for a parametric survival model. *Journal of the Royal Statistical Society, Series B*, **58**, 417–424.

Crowder, M. (1997). A test for independence of competing risks with discrete failure times. *Lifetime Data Analysis*, **3**, 215–223.

Crowder, M. (2001) *Classical Competing Risks*. Boca Raton, FL: Chapman & Hall/CRC.

David, H. A. and Moeschberger, M. L. (1978) *The Theory of Competing Risks*. London: Griffin.

Dewan, I., Deshpande, J. V. and Kulathinal, S. B. (2004). On testing dependence between time to failure and cause of failure via conditional probabilities. *Scandinavian Journal of Statistics*, **31**, 79–91.

Dinse, G. E. and Larson, M. G. (1986). A note on semi-Markov models for partially censored data. *Biometrika*, **73**, 379–386.

Efron, B. (1977). Efficiency of Cox's likelihood function for censored data. *Journal of the American Statistical Association*, **72**, 557–565.

Feller, W. (1951). The asymptotic distribution of the range of sums of independent random variables. *Annals of Mathematical Statistics*, **22**, 427–432.

Fine, J. P. (1999). Analysing competing risks data with transformation models. *Journal of the Royal Statistical Society, Series B*, **61**, 817–830.

Fine, J. P. and Gray, R. J. (1999). A proportional hazards model for the subdistribution of a competing risk. *Journal of the Americal Statistical Association*, **94**, 496–509.

Fox, J. (2002) *An R and S-PLUS Companion to Applied Regression*. Thousand Oaks, CA: Sage.

Fyles, A., Milosevic, M., Hedley, D., Pintilie, M., Levin, W., Manchul, L. and Hill, R. P. (2002). Tumor hypoxia has independent predictor impact only in patients with node-negative cervix cancer. *Journal of Clinical Oncology*, **20**, 680–687.

Fyles, A. W., McCready, D. R., Manchul, L. A., Trudeau, M. E., Merante, P., Pintilie, M., Weir, L. M. and Olivotto, I. A. (2004). Tamoxifen with or without breast irradiation in women 50 years of age or older with early breast cancer. *New England Journal of Medicine*, **351**, 963–970.

Gaynor, J. J., Feuer, E. J., Tan, C. C., Wu, D. H., Little, C. R., Straus, D. J., Clarkson, B. D. and Brennan, M. F. (1993). On the use of cause-specific failure and conditional failure probabilities – examples from clinical oncology data. *Journal of the American Statistical Association,* **88**, 400–409.

Gelman, R., Gelber, R., Henderson, I. C., Coleman, C. N. and Harris, J. R. (1990). Improved methodology for analyzing local and distant recurrence. *Journal of Clinical Oncology,* **8**, 548–555.

Gooley, T. A., Leisenring, W., Crowley, J. and Storer, B. E. (1999). Estimation of failure probabilities in the presence of competing risks: new representations of old estimators. *Statistics in Medicine,* **18**, 695–706.

Graunt, J. (1662) *Natural and political observations, mentioned in a following Index, and made upon the Bills of Mortality.* London: Tho. Roycroft.

Gray, R. J. (1988). A class of *k*-sample tests for comparing the cumulative incidence of a competing risk. *Annals of Statistics,* **16**, 1141–1154.

Hall, W. J. and Wellner, J. A. (1980). Confidence bands for a survival curve from censored data. *Biometrika,* **67**, 133–143.

Halley, E. (1693). An estimate of the degrees of the mortality of mankind, drawn from curious tables of the births and funerals at the city of Breslaw. *Philosophical Transactions of the Royal Society of London,* **17**, 596–610.

Kalbfleisch, J. D. and Prentice, R. L. (1980) *The Statistical Analysis of Failure Time Data.* New York: John Wiley & Sons, Inc.

Kalbfleisch, J. D. and Prentice, R. L. (2002) *The Statistical Analysis of Failure Time Data.* Hoboken, NJ: John Wiley & Sons, Inc.

Kaplan, E. L. and Meier, P. (1958). Nonparametric estimation from incomplete observations. *Journal of the American Statistical Association,* **53**, 457–481.

Kochar, S. C., Lam, K. F. and Yip, P. S. F. (2002). Generalized supremum tests for the equality of cause specific hazard rates. *Lifetime Data Analysis,* **8**, 277–288.

Korn, E. L. and Dorey, F. J. (1992). Applications of crude incidence curves. *Statistics in Medicine,* **11**, 813–829.

Kulathinal, S. B. and Gasbarra, D. (2002). Testing equality of cause-specific hazard rates corresponding to *m* competing risks among *k* groups. *Lifetime Data Analysis,* **8**, 147–161.

Larson, M. G. and Dinse, G. E. (1985). A mixture model for the regression analysis of competing risks data. *Applied Statistics,* **34**, 201–211.

Lawless, J. F. (1982) *Statistical Models and Methods for Lifetime Data.* New York: John Wiley & Sons, Inc.

Lin, D. Y. (1997). Non-parametric inference for cumulative incidence functions in competing risks studies. *Statistics in Medicine,* **16**, 901–910.

Lin, D. Y., Robins, J. M. and Wei, L. J. (1996). Comparing two failure time distributions in the presence of dependent censoring. *Biometrika,* **83**, 381–393.

Lunn, M. (1998). Applying k-sample tests to conditional probabilities for competing risks in a clinical trial. *Biometrics*, **54**, 1662–1672.

Maller, R. A. and Zhou, X. (2002). Analysis of parametric models for competing risks. *Statistica Sinica*, **12**, 725–750.

Marubini, E. and Valsecchi, M. (1995) *Analysing Survival Data from Clinical Trials and Observational Studies*. Chichester: John Wiley & Sons, Ltd.

Matthews, D. E. (1988). Likelihood-based confidence intervals for functions of many parameters. *Biometrika*. **75**, 139–144.

Milosevic, M. F., Fyles, A. W., Wong, R., Pintilie, M., Kavanagh, M. C., Levin, W., Manchul, L. A., Keane, T. J. and Hill, R. P. (1998). Interstitial fluid pressure in cervical carcinoma: within tumor heterogeneity, and relation to oxygen tension. *Cancer*, **82**, 2418–2426.

Milosevic, M., Fyles, A., Hedley, D., Pintilie, M., Levin, W., Manchul, L. and Hill, R. (2001). Interstitial fluid pressure predicts survival in patients with cervix cancer independent of clinical prognostic factors and tumor oxygen measurements. *Cancer Research*, **61**, 6400–6405.

Nelson, W. (1972). Theory and applications of hazard plotting for censored failure data. *Technometrics*, **14**, 945–965.

Pepe, M. S. (1991). Inference for events with dependent risks in multiple endpoint studies. *Journal of the American Statistical Association*, **86**, 770–778.

Pepe, M. S. and Fleming, T. R. (1991) Weighted Kaplan–Meier statistics: Large sample and optimality considerations. *Journal of the Royal Statistical Society, Series B*, **53**, 341–352.

Pepe, M. S. and Mori, M. (1993). Kaplan–Meier, marginal or conditional probability curves in summarizing competing risks failure time data? *Statistics in Medicine*, **12**, 737–751.

Petersen, P., Tsang, R., Gospodarowicz, M., Pintilie, M., Wells, W., Hodgson, D., Sun, A. and Crump, M. (2004a). Stage I and II Hodgkin's disease: Long term outcome and second cancer risk. *Radiotherapy and Oncology*, **72**, S23.

Petersen, P. M., Gospodarowicz, M., Tsang, R., Pintilie, M., Wells, W., Hodgson, D., Sun, A., Crump, M., Patterson, B. and Bailey, D. (2004b). Long-term outcome in stage I and II follicular lymphoma following treatment with involved field radiation therapy alone. *Journal of Clinical Oncology*, **22**, 563S.

Pintilie, M. (2002). Dealing with competing risks: testing covariates and calculating sample size. *Statistics in Medicine*, **21**, 3317–3324.

Rowe, P. J., Boccard, S., Farley, T. M. M., Peregoudov, S., Reinprayoon, D., Koetsawang, S., Wu, S. C., Gopalan, S., Xiem, N. T., de la Concepción, O., Andolsek-Jeras, L., Sikazwe, N. C., Ramos, R. M., Dubnitskaya, L., Pizarro, E., Grimon, R. U., Cardet, E. C., Zhuang, L. Q., Fen, W. Y., Hao, W. Y., McCarthy, T., Nikanorova, S., Bartfai, G., Khodjaeva, R. K.,

Boukhris, M. M., Wu, X. R. and Aroustamian, K. (1997). Long-term reversible contraception. Twelve years of experience with the TCu380A and TCu220C. *Contraception.* **56**, 341–352.

Scrutinio, D., Cimminiello, C., Marubini, E., Pitzalis, M. V., Di Biase, M. and Rizzon, P. (2001). Ticlopidine versus aspirin after myocardial infarction (STAMI) trial. *Journal of the American College of Cardiology,* **37**, 1259–1265.

Tai, B.-C., Peregoudov, A. and Machin, D. (2001). A competing risk approach to the analysis of trials of alternative intra-uterine devices (IUDs) for fertility regulation. *Statistics in Medicine,* **20**, 3589–3600.

Tai, B.-C., White, I. R., Gebski, V. and Machin, D. (2002). On the issue of 'multiple' first failures in competing risks analysis. *Statistics in Medicine,* **21**, 2243–2255.

Therneau, T. and Grambsch, P. (2000) *Modeling Survival Data: Extending the Cox Model.* New York: Springer-Verlag.

Tsiatis, A. (1975). A nonidentifiability aspect of the problem of competing risks. *Proceedings of the National Academy of Sciences of the United States of America,* **72**, 20–22.

Wong, R. K. W., Fyles, A., Milosevic, M., Pintilie, M. and Hill, R. P. (1997). Heterogeneity of polarographic oxygen tension measurements in cervix cancer: An evaluation of within and between tumor variability, probe position, and track depth. *International Journal of Radiation Oncology, Biology, Physics,* **39**, 405–412.

Index

Page references in **bold** refer to tables, page references in *italics* refer to figures

Competing Risks: A Practical Perspective   M. Pintilie
© 2006 John Wiley & Sons, Ltd

Printed and bound by CPI Group (UK) Ltd, Croydon, CR0 4YY

27/10/2024

14580207-0002